FOURTEEN FRIENDS'
GUIDE TO
ELDERCARING

PRACTICAL ADVICE

❧

INSPIRATION

❧

SHARED EXPERIENCES

❧

SPACE FOR YOUR THOUGHTS

Published by
Capital Books Inc.
22883 Quicksilver Drive
Sterling, Virginia 20166
Printed in Hong Kong through PrintNet

Attention Organizations:

CAPITAL BOOKS are available at quantity discounts with
bulk purchase for educational, business, or sales promotional
use. For information, please write to: SPECIAL SALES
DEPARTMENT, Capital Books, P.O. Box 605, Herndon,
Virginia 20172-0605 or call TOLL FREE 1-800-758-3756.

Library of Congress Cataloging-in-Publication Data

Fourteen Friends' guide to eldercaring : practical advice,
inspiration, shared experiences, space for your thoughts /
written by the Fourteen Friends, Joan Hunter Cooper …
[et al.] ; with photographs and illustrations by Judy
Sherwood McLeod and friends.
     p. cm.
   Includes bibliographical references.
   ISBN 1-892123-08-8
   1. Aged—Care—United States. 2. Aged—United States—
Psychology. 3. Caregivers—United States—Psychology.
   4. Caregivers—United States—Attitudes.
   I. Cooper, Joan Hunter. II. Title: Eldercaring.
HQ1064.U5F635 1999
362.6'0973—dc21

NOTE: This book is an adjunct to, not a substitute for,
conventional medical therapy and legal advice. For major
decisions affecting your own health and legal issues or
those of someone for whom you care, please consult your
physician or attorney.

Produced by Judd Publishing, Inc.
Designed by Caroline Brock

FOURTEEN FRIENDS'
GUIDE TO
ELDERCARING

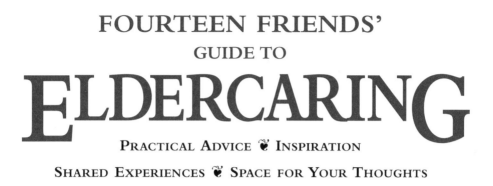

PRACTICAL ADVICE ❦ INSPIRATION

SHARED EXPERIENCES ❦ SPACE FOR YOUR THOUGHTS

Written by the Fourteen Friends:

Joan Hunter Cooper
Judy Fulton Guerin
Joan Berkey Loftis
Alice Beckley MacDonald
Judy Sherwood McLeod
Beth Sanders Milner
Lee Lambie Pope
Anne Smith Roadman
Linda Gilbertson Rogers
Karen Wulfsberg Strother
Karen Kelley Thalinger, MD
Linda Staley Veatch
Brenda Jones Vieregg
Carol Cummings Warner

With Photographs and Illustrations by
Judy Sherwood McLeod
and Friends

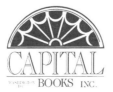

CAPITAL
BOOKS INC.

CONTENTS

you and your time will become more manageable when you are flexible.

Frustration is normal and inevitable. Find solace in humor and in education. Recognizing and accepting the things that cannot be changed will relieve stress.

Recognize that the mental well-being of the caregiver benefits everyone involved. An overworked, stressed-out caregiver will not be able to give quality care.

Long distance eldercaring presents special challenges for the caregiver. Establish and use a network of assistance in the locale of the elder as well as support in the locale of the caregiver.

Ways are suggested to preserve your aging loved one's dignity for a happier person and a more compatible relationship with you, the caregiver. Remember that someday we may be in the same position.

How to recognize the inevitable changes in brain functioning in your elders.

A list of where to go for services, support and other related necessities, and whom to ask for help.

Names, addresses, and information to make this journal a "support group" in itself by adding to the information provided.

Fourteen Friends is an extraordinary support group; it is not listed in the yellow pages, or in any health agency's catalogue. We are not a group of experts. We are fourteen girlfriends, now living in six different states and the District of Columbia, who have known each other since childhood. We have shared ideas and experiences about school, marriage, children, divorce, and careers, during happy times and sad times. As women and mothers, we are a diverse group: a neurologist, a psychiatric nurse practitioner, an accountant, a counselor, an artist (who has done all the artwork and most of the photography for this journal), educators and businesswomen. Several years ago at our regular get-togethers the topic of conversation gradually switched from raising children to caring for parents.

Eldercaring has since become our most challenging role. Sharing with each other has given us strength and has deepened our understanding of the challenges each of us is facing. More than anything else, sharing with each other made us want to share with you, the reader, the experience of what we now call "Eldercaring." We hope this will be the first of our Fourteen Friends' guides to caring and care giving.

Almost everyone is a caregiver at some point in his or her life. Anyone caught in the "sandwich" generation may be giving care to two generations: the younger one to whom they gave life, and the older one that gave life to them. This now middle-aged generation will find this book particularly beneficial. As a part of the 22.5 million caregivers in the nation today, we, the authors, share firsthand knowledge of care giving for our own aging relatives — some of whom are suffering from a variety of ailments including Alzheimer's Disease, stroke, Parkinson's Disease, alcoholism, heart disease, cancer, macular degeneration, arthritis and dementia.

> *Friends are an aid to the young, to guard them from error; to the elderly, to attend to their wants and to supplement their failing power of action; to those in the prime of life, to assist them to noble deeds.*
>
> — Aristotle, *Thoughts on Success* (Chicago: Triumph Books, 1995, p. 73)

You will find that *Eldercaring* is not just for dealing with illness. We intend it to be a useful guide for all aspects of eldercaring; useful for helping parents cope with changes in their lifestyle; useful for anyone frustrated in their attempts to help someone else through difficult times. By passing along our individual and collective experiences, research and suggestions, we hope you will discover new perspectives and solutions to the challenges you may encounter along your own journey. Our wish is that this journal will make your eldercaring more manageable and less stressful.

It is not essential that you have an "elder" to find this book helpful. It has universal themes involved in care giving such as guilt, frustration and flexibility. You will use it the minute you leave the doctor's office and realize you didn't have time to discuss 90 percent of the problems you should have addressed. Eldercaring is intended to help you get the most out of all the support services available, for both the caregiver and the recipient of care.

The demands of eldercaring are great — and change daily. This journal is set up so you can find relevant, helpful and inspirational information. The planner will help you keep track of schedules, activities and appointments. There are eldercaring tips as well as reflective quotes and space to record your day-to-day observations, personal thoughts or ideas. Forms are provided for telephone numbers and addresses, medications and other essential information. We have designed our journal to be easily used and carried with you, so you have necessary phone numbers and vital information no matter when the need arises.

Please carry, also, our good wishes.

Joan Hunter Cooper
Dallas, Texas
Judy Fulton Guerin
Paradise Valley, Arizona
Joan Berkey Loftis
Arlington, Virginia
Alice Beckley MacDonald
Herndon, Virginia
Judy Sherwood McLeod
Charlottesville, Virginia
Beth Sanders Milner
Middleburg, Virginia
Lee Lambie Pope
Point Pleasant, New Jersey
Anne Smith Roadman
Washington, D.C.
Linda Gilbertson Rogers
Arlington, Virginia
Karen Wulfsberg Strother
Lone Tree, Colorado
Karen Kelley Thalinger, MD
Ponte Vedra Beach, Florida
Linda Staley Veatch
Oakton, Virginia
Brenda Jones Viereg
Fairfax, Virginia
Carol Cummings Warner
Washington, D.C.

Nearby travelers at the Colorado Springs Airport could not help but notice the obvious excitement — the hugs, the chatter and laughter as the Fourteen Friends, with luggage in hand, gathered after the planes arrived from various cities across the U.S. We were about to spend five days together hiking, white-water rafting, catching up with the latest family and career news and sharing ideas. This was not our first gathering; for the past ten years we had been meeting annually at the beach. Because of our different backgrounds and directions since high school, we had helped each other understand problems from different perspectives. The annual get-together usually included a presentation by one of the group on topics ranging from Fabergé eggs to fractals, breast exams to brain functioning. Conversation continued on the beach. Through sharing, we each left with a greater understanding of our own challenges and ways to meet them.

DIFFICULT DECISIONS, DIFFICULT CHANGES

Understanding our aging loved ones and helping others to understand is the first step to successful care giving.

This involves many facets:

• Understanding the reasons why an older family member is in need of help

• Understanding the emotions of an aging loved one

• Understanding the feelings and emotions of the family unit as a whole and as individuals

• Understanding our own personal emotions.

Difficult decisions, difficult choices, and difficult changes all have to be made as aging of a loved one progresses.

UNDERSTANDING

Mistakes will be avoided when enough time is devoted to tolerance and sympathy. Understanding should be the first step for caregivers.

The external signs of aging require little explanation. More difficult to understand and recognize are the internal changes occurring in all the body's systems, not the least of which is the brain. It is tempting to think that the brain is unaffected by disturbances in other parts of the body, but the brain thrives on a proper environment of adequate blood flow, oxygen and glucose. With aging, the brain is less tolerant of fluctuations in these areas because it has lost some of its reserve

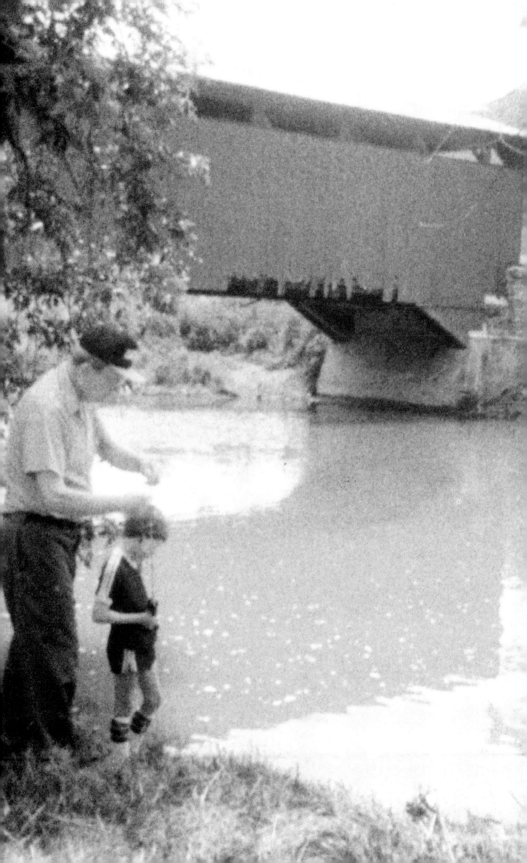

forces and its ability to rebound. Even mentally alert older people can become delirious or emotionally unstable when they have illnesses such as pneumonia, heart disease or other common conditions. This may cause the normally rational, cooperative person to become like an unreasonable "child." Patients with dementia, whether due to Alzheimer's Disease, strokes, or other serious conditions, are even more vulnerable to the effects of illness. As caregivers, it is of primary importance to understand these physical and emotional relationships.

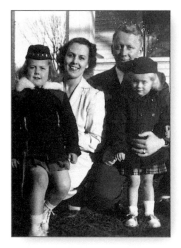

Understanding the complexity of emotions of an older family member is yet another challenge for the caregiver. Generational gaps are unavoidable; an aging loved one and caregivers will perceive or react to issues differently. What was "proper" in their parents' household and what was expected in their generation may create anxiety and resistance in the caregiver. For example, the loved ones may refuse to be bathed because of modesty issues that were part of their upbringing. Re-examining and acknowledging generational differences will help in creating solutions.

OPEN COMMUNICATION PROMOTES UNDERSTANDING

Eldercaring is often a shared responsibility, and this requires understanding each person's unique point of view. Dialogue, consideration and cooperation are critical. Fellow caregivers may show anger, resentment, and inconsistency. Some may insist on carrying all the responsibility or conversely, may be unable to bear much responsibility at all. It is important to strive to understand the source of and reasons for the various responses and personal feelings. It is not possible for all caregivers to react and respond in exactly the same way. Examine each caregiver's strengths and capitalize on them! Open communication promotes understanding.

Caregivers need to understand the impact of eldercaring on themselves. Personal limitations and personal needs are frequently neglected by the caregiver. Overextending to the point of exhaustion and poor health creates difficulties rather than solutions.

Finally, a critical part in this initial step is helping others to understand. Professional caregivers such as home companions, day-care staffers, or a medical provider will be more considerate and effective when time is dedicated to teaching them about the unique personality and preferences of an aging loved one.

> *Understanding is the antidote for frustration.*

BREAKING THE CODE

Try to discover why your elder reacts as he does. Is there a hidden issue underlying his words and actions? You may be surprised to find that:

- "I don't want to do that" may mean I can't do that anymore.
- "I don't want steak" may mean I can't cut it or chew it.
- "I don't want to go" may mean it's too far from a bathroom, or too far to walk, or has too many steps.
- "I don't want to go shopping at the mall" may mean it's too much walking (take a "courtesy" wheelchair and save energy for shopping in the stores).

Notes

ELDERCARING IS LIKE TENDING A GARDEN

"Tending a garden is a natural metaphor for cultivating an inner life. The art of cultivating…can nurture the landscape of our lives, transforming a barren survival into a fruitful existence."

— Cathleen Rountree,
On Women Turning 50
(New York: Harper Collins, 1993, p. 9)

My friend's mother had a series of falls and operations which caused her to be in and out of the hospital. Each time another crisis occurred, she said, "Don't tell anyone that I'm in the hospital." I couldn't understand why she insisted on secrecy until a former colleague gave a graduation address and spoke about the difficulty he had accepting help with his own terminal disease.

Like him, my friend's mother didn't want to feel dependent and, in her case, old. But that kept her from being helped and loved by those who wanted to do anything they could for her. We have been taught to give, but learning to receive help is often difficult.

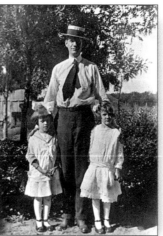

♥ TIPS FOR CARE GIVING

♥ Be early, not late. You can be five minutes early but never five minutes late! Time has a different meaning for the elderly. Planning ahead will prevent frustration on your part and anxiety for the elder.

♥ Little things become big. Small issues to you may be important to them. Accept that their world could narrow to only those things that directly affect them: their pain, their discomfort, their visitors, their losses, their fear, their failing bodies. This more limited world view may prevent them from listening and responding to the needs and activities of anyone else and may make it difficult to carry on a two-way conversation.

♥ Don't focus on outward behavior. Analyze the inner reason.

♥ Life can only be understood backwards. But it must be lived forwards.

♥ Understand that no one is perfect.

Notes

> "I want,
> by understanding
> myself, to understand
> others. I want to be
> all that I am
> capable of becoming. "
>
> — Katherine Mansfield

CUT THE WHEAT FROM THE CHAFF

Try to determine quickly what really matters. Avoid sidetracks and pay attention to the essentials. Caregivers should alert the physician to any sudden deterioration of health so that correctable problems can be addressed. Be aware of changes in personality as well and use this book to make a note of their development so you can answer questions about the onset of problems. The diagnosis of a chronic, incurable illness should not deter you from seeking further help. If you are told, "Nothing more can be done," seek a second opinion. Measures to comfort the patient and ease the burdens of the caregiver are always available and may be as simple as an adjustment in medication.

"No act of kindness, no matter how small, is ever wasted."

— *Aesop's Fables*

"I've learned that regardless of how little you have, you can always give comfort and encouragement."

— H. Jackson Brown, Jr.,
Live & Learn & Pass It On
(Nashville: Rutledge
Hill Press, Inc., 1991, p. 110)

"Never miss a chance to keep your mouth shut."

— Robert Newton Peck

An Exercise

Understand upbringing
Understand personality
Understand loss of control
Understand impact on family
Understand professional advice
Understand your own resistance.

"I've learned that the great challenge of life is to decide what's important and to disregard everything else."

— H. Jackson Brown, Jr.,
Live and Learn and Pass it On
(Ibid, p. 14)

REMEMBER — you catch more flies with honey than with vinegar!

"What you see and hear depends a good deal on where you are standing; it also depends on what sort of person you are."

— C.S. Lewis,
The Magician's Nephew

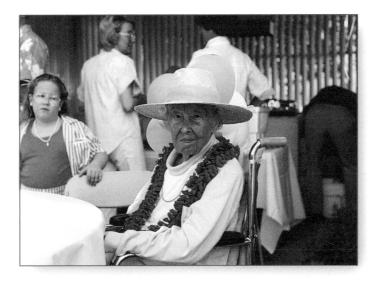

"What Part of What I Said Do You Not Understand?!"

My parents who live six hours away from me frequently complain that my sister and I don't visit often enough. Every phone conversation with my mother begins and ends with, "When are you coming to see us? Please come visit anytime." Recently, I called two weeks ahead to let her know that my sister and I and our spouses would be coming to celebrate her eighty-fifth birthday. I made it very clear that we would arrive Friday night and leave Sunday morning.

Instead of the delighted response I expected, I heard hesitation and worry. Mother immediately started talking about a dinner party and a brunch that they were attending on Sunday. I reiterated that we would have left by then but had to discuss these possible conflicts twice more during the conversation.

After expressing my irritation to my husband, he reminded me that older people don't always process information as quickly as they once did. They may become overwhelmed by too much information. In the future I won't ask for an immediate answer.

I can also understand that coming on a different weekend would have made her birthday celebration last longer. Probably many week-ends have no activities at all. This one had too many!

"The American dilemma, at the century's close, is what to do about the hidden costs of longevity — not just the economic ones, but the intimate, personal costs as well."

— Ted Conover, "The Last Best Friends Money Can Buy"
(*The New York Times Magazine*, November 30, 1997, p. 132)

❤ MORE TIPS FOR CARE GIVING

❤ Patience is paramount. Plan ahead yet be prepared to change course midstream. Be flexible in your responses. With a flexible outlook, demands that seem irrational may become manageable.

❤ Don't judge! If you criticize your fellow caregivers, you may end up with the whole job. Communicate with each other and always listen carefully for underlying messages.

❤ Be compassionate. Picture yourself in the position of the elder to better understand the situation. It isn't easy to constantly be needing help.

❤ Manipulation is a two-way process. Loss of control creates the desire to control something or someone else. Understand underlying reasons to avoid anger and the temptation to retaliate.

Notes

> *"Time waits for no one. Treasure every moment you have. You will treasure it even more when you can share it with someone special."*
>
> — Ann Landers
> (*The Washington Post*, February 26, 1998)

N o t e s

During a recent office visit, one of my Alzheimer's Disease patients and his wife told me about their trip to New Orleans to celebrate their 54th wedding anniversary. As his wife checked in at the airport and got the boarding passes, she commented to the ticket clerk that her husband had Alzheimer's Disease and they were taking the anniversary trip while he could still enjoy it. The clerk asked to have the boarding passes back and reseated them in First Class! They were thrilled.

ENCOURAGEMENT

the fullest within the boundaries of their physical limitations will be achieved through realistic expectations. If they can't do more, a simple routine of walking up and down the halls rather than around the block, or learning to exercise and stretch in a chair rather than not walking at all will elevate their spirits. Music therapy works too! As caregivers we may enjoy revisiting the music of the 1960s and 1970s. Offer your elder music from their own favorite era.

BE ENCOURAGED BY RANDOM ACTS OF KINDNESS

Keeping an older loved one's spirits lively is a vital part of eldercaring. Expectations can play a major role in the encouragement you provide for your elder. The idea of "self-fulfilling prophecy" is so apparent: People become what is expected of them regardless of age or health. When you set loving expectations and make small adjustments, you give self-respect and personal satisfaction to an older, dependent person.

KEEPING SPIRITS LIVELY

Helping our elderly discover ways of continuing to live life to

In the areas of personal grooming and appearance, older people need gentle help. Encourage good personal grooming with regular attention to hair cuts and styling, makeup, and attractive, clean and comfortable clothing. Make it fun — give them a manicure. When appropriate, interest your loved ones in improving their surroundings with cheerful colors, plants, or flowers. Special aromas also can encourage better feelings.

Another successful strategy for wellbeing is pet therapy. One Alzheimer's patient always brightened up when talking about his dog Ginger. Taking a pet to visit your elder may brighten the day.

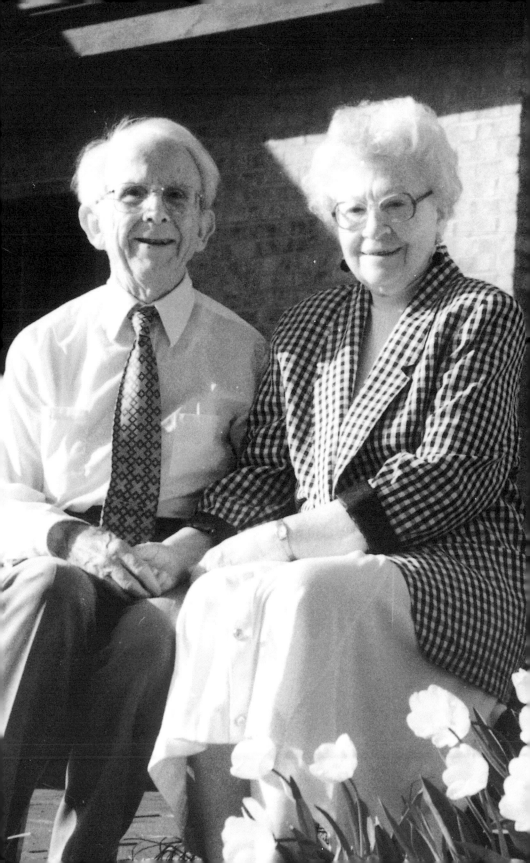

Whenever possible, encourage your loved one's active participation in daily routines.

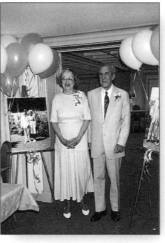

Maintenance of self-esteem enhances senescence, the process of growing old. Self-esteem is elevated through interaction with people. A warm relationship with the caregiver can allow dependence to be friendship rather than burden. Changes in physical and mental well-being may lead to isolation and depression. The caregiver can provide opportunities for interaction with people in the community. One stroke patient who cannot speak and lives on a busy street loves to sit in her bay window. The interesting street life keeps her entertained for hours as she waves to friends and keeps track of all the action.

As a caregiver, recollect what things were most important to your loved one before, and you will deal better with the present situation and its limitations. What was important? Social status? Friendships? Family? Independence? Intellect? Physical activity? Bridge games? Hobbies? Things that were not important before will not become so now just because you, the caregiver, wish they would. You cannot expect the person being cared for to be someone they haven't been. Encourage what they always have enjoyed and help them to maintain the best parts of their personal dignity.

Open discussions with friends and family members about your loved one's previous interests and personality characteristics will help everyone give encouragement and set expectations. Understanding threads deeply into the activity of encouragement. Remember, an essential ingredient of a good life is a strong spirit. Encourage it.

> *Encouragement is the antidote for hesitation.*

❤ Tips for Caregivers

❤ Don't give up too soon. *I was encouraged that after having another one-sided conversation with my mother, an Alzheimer's patient, she responded with a whole sentence!* You cannot assume that what you say is not being understood just because at times there appears to be little response.

❤ Take small steps. *I was frustrated that things I was doing did not seem to help. Then I realized that tiny little steps were better than none.*

❤ Keep a camera handy. Everyone cares how they look, no matter how old they are. Taking their picture because they look so nice will encourage grooming as will a weekly excursion they can dress for and anticipate.

❤ Encourage goal setting. Help identify enjoyable events which will also be beneficial physically. *An elderly acquaintance started walking the block to the grocery store every day to convince her family that she was physically capable of flying across the country alone to visit a gentleman friend. When the purpose had been just exercise, she wasn't interested; when it was connected to a goal of her choosing, she worked very hard!*

❤ Avoid isolation. In assisted living facilities, suite living where elderly people have a private bedroom but share at least a living room can be better than private quarters. If they have just given up their homes, adjustment to a lack of privacy is difficult, but together suite mates can share complaints, urge each other on and lift each other's spirits.

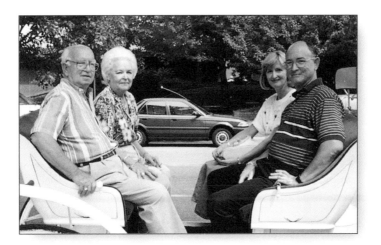

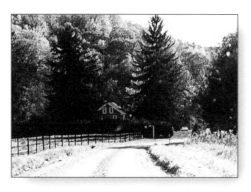

"You must do the thing you think you cannot do."

— Eleanor Roosevelt

In the last few days of my mother's life, her best-loved older brother and his wonderful wife arrived with other family members for our final farewells. After an extremely difficult night, my mother briefly gained coherence, clarity, and vision. With special loving words for each person, she was at peace, and let life go. A few minutes later my elderly aunt gave me profound and life-long comfort when, placing her hand on my arm she said, "It's okay and right for you to miss her. My own mother died 58 YEARS AGO and I still miss her." This set me free.

LET RESEARCH WORK FOR YOU

Get on the mailing list for the newsletters of associations like the Alzheimer's Association. It is encouraging that research is constantly making revelations that are helpful to both the caregiver and the elder. Here are a few examples:

• Counseling Support

"A recent study by New York researchers found that when spouses caring for Alzheimer's patients took part in a counseling and support program, institutional placement was delayed by nearly a year."

— *Harvard Health Letter* (February 1997, vol. 22, p. 8)

• Benefits Of Exercise

"All those mall walkers are on to something: A major study found that a daily stroll keeps older people living longer."

— *The Washington Post* (January 8, 1998, p. A10.)

• Physical Environment

"Like birth, aging is a process, not an illness; therefore, a physical environment for older people must be designed to celebrate life, promote health and wellness, enhance the abilities of older adults, and encourage social interaction with friends, family ties, staff, and the community at large. A transformation of the nursing home into this kind of environment will benefit everyone involved in longterm care."

— "The Nursing Home Revisited," by Eunice Noell, *Generations* (Winter 1995, vol. 19, p. 14).

HAVE FUN!

My parents are fortunate to live in a retirement facility in Virginia where many professional people from varied backgrounds reside. These people stay busy with clubs, cards and many special programs. Their latest fad is betting on horses with play money. It's a fun activity (highly organized by them) and they share hosting duties for different races. This involves bringing food for a pregame cocktail party. Planning and participating in these events keeps them alive and lively, not to mention very much connected with each other.

NEVER SAY NEVER

What is right for one person won't work for another. One person's negative is another person's positive. Weigh the pluses and the minuses. Once you've made the decision, don't look back. What you decided is right for the moment but change is imminent. The only thing you can count on is change.

You're not alone! Consult friends, relatives, and professionals for help. Ask your doctor if a home health evaluation can be prescribed to determine the need for eligible services such as physical therapy or home health aides which would be covered by Medicare.

Notes

TOUCH!

There may be no words that can make an elderly or ill person feel better, but your touch can make them feel that you care in a way that words and deeds do not. A hug, a pat on the shoulder or holding their hand can bring great solace. It may provide the encouragement needed to complete a difficult task or just get through a gloomy hour. After a long, close marriage filled with physical affection, a widow may go for weeks, even months, without being touched by another person! One reason that pets raise our spirits is that we touch them and they nuzzle back. *When talking about her husband and explaining why she loves him, a young woman gives an example that whenever he is in the room with his grandmother, he holds her hand.* That kind of touching does not come naturally to everyone, but when it does it can compete with most of the medicine that elderly people receive!

Perhaps the lack of touch is one reason the elderly often ask to take someone's arm. They are not only concerned about falling; they enjoy the sense of physical closeness to another person, and it's an acceptable way to ask for it. If you are not comfortable just sitting and holding someone's hand, try touching their back when they go through a door or just touching their hand when you greet them and say goodbye.

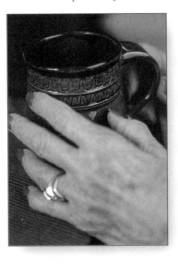

Trying to think of a gift that might make a difference? Give a massage, a manicure or a pedicure. The greatest value may not be in the grooming but the touch. Or give a certificate to have these services performed. While not the hands of a friend or loved one, the touch is still valuable, not quite so personal but touch just the same!

> *"Let me be a little kinder, Let me be a little blinder, To the faults of those around me, Let me praise a little more."*
>
> — Edgar Albert Guest,
> *A Creed*

N o t e s

> "*Praise is the best diet for us, after all.*"
>
> — Sydney Smith,
> *Lady Holland's Memoir*

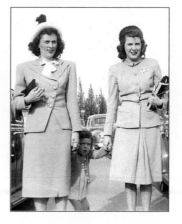

Noah contemplated whether Allie, suffering with Alzheimer's, would respond: *"I wonder, will it happen today? I don't know, for I never know beforehand, and deep down it really doesn't matter. It's the possibility that keeps me going, not the guarantee, a sort of wager on my part. And though you may call me a dreamer or fool or any other thing, I believe that anything is possible."*

— Nicholas Sparks,
The Notebook (New York:
Warner Books, Inc., 1996, p. 5)

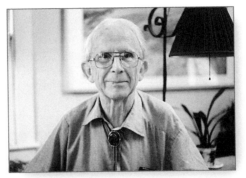

CAREGIVERS THEMSELVES

Having the opportunity to take part in caring for others can encourage the elderly to feel that life is worthwhile because they are still needed.

Feeling that she is encouraging others makes my mother-in-law feel useful and important. Her most important roles in life were as nurse, wife and parent, and nurturing makes her happy. When she went to a retirement home, what she missed most of all were her dogs and the birds she had fed every day. They were the last of a list of things that she had cared for and now lost — her child had grown up, her husband died and finally she had been removed from her pets. She wanted to feel that she could still give, as well as receive, care.

Some retirement facilities allow pets. Nurturing can be of a dog or cat, a bird or fish. An aquarium can provide the routine and responsibility of feeding, as well as the serenity that comes from watching them.

Tending can even be to a plant. Just as forcing bulbs during the winter gives you a lift, they can be rewarding and inspiring to the

"It has always been so: That sign of old age — extolling the past at the expense of the present."

— Sydney Smith,
Lady Holland's Memoir

elderly. You can almost see them grow before your eyes and progress is a scarce commodity for the aging!

The elderly can reap the bene- fit of caring for each other. One woman was encouraged by helping a recently widowed friend participate after isolating herself following her husband's death.

Notes

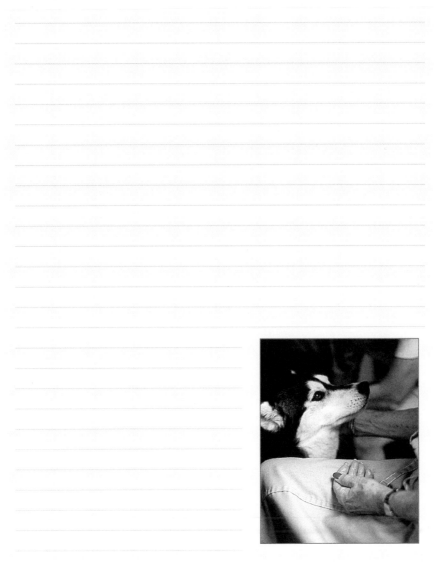

*W*e call our Aunt Rosie *"Alexandra Haig." "I'm in charge here"* were the first words out of her mouth when the family all gathered after my father had a debilitating stroke. And in charge she was because she had been given my father's power of attorney. Good, we thought; she can handle the bills and insurance. Little did we know, however, that SHE alone was going to decide and orchestrate what she thought was best for my father for the rest of his life. She rejected any initial advice or suggestions, and therefore she got no help. She continues to make all the decisions, handles all the doctor appointments, pays all the bills, the insurance and taxes, hires and fires the live-in caregivers, maintains my father's apartment and garden; handles the Christmas decorations and the cat. She is frustrated and overworked most of the time but can't understand why she gets no help. If there were ever a scenario of what not to do in care giving, that is it in a nutshell.

MOST JOBS ARE EASIER WHEN SHARED

Eldercaring is a tough job. Most jobs are easier when they can be shared. Sharing eldercaring is especially difficult because of all the emotions and personalities involved.

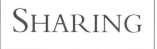

Though each caregiver may be well meaning, there will be varying opinions about how to handle the situation.

Sharing eldercaring must include sharing time and physical requirements, sharing medical and legal decision-making, and meeting the emotional needs of the dependent. A caregiver who tries to handle all of these responsibilities alone will be physically and emotionally depleted and thereby ineffective. Involving as many caregivers as possible will lighten the load. Cooperation among all will make the eldercaring more satisfying and less stressful for everyone.

Early on, make a list of all areas where help is needed. Acknowledge what are the essential requirements and what are the added niceties. Determine and assess how each caregiver is willing and able to participate. Capitalize on each person's strengths and abilities and don't ask the impossible. Divide the responsibilities accordingly. You can't expect someone with a full-time job to handle the daytime doctor appointments, and you don't expect someone who lives an hour away to make daily visits. Each caregiver's tasks may be different and not necessarily

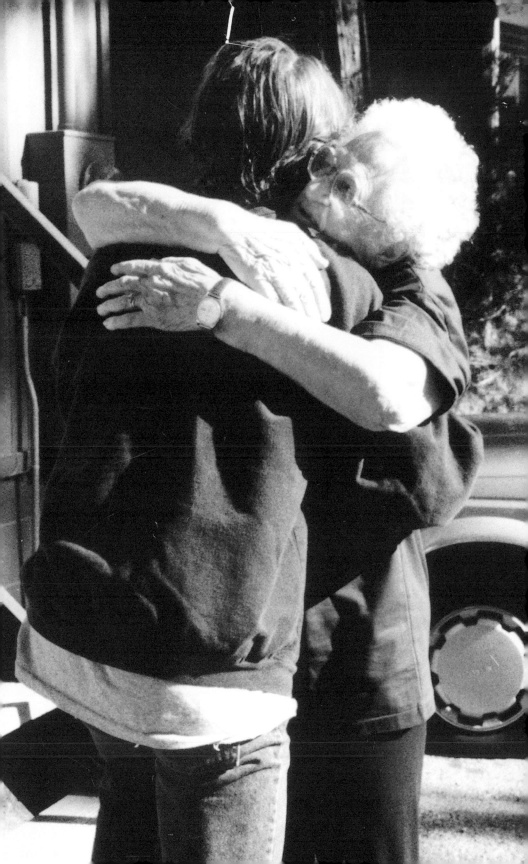

equal. It may not turn out to be fair.

Care giving can be shared with organizations outside the home. There are many senior centers with adult day care programs available, some of which even provide transportation. These day care centers provide companionship, an important ingredient for active minds and healthy bodies. There are many support groups that can suggest resources and offer practical help that are specific to a particular disease or disability. Many churches have volunteers available to aid homebound people with their needs. Agencies like Meals on Wheels can be the lifesaver that allows a person to remain in his home. Some grocery stores have order and delivery service — some will bill the customer who cannot handle cash. A little research in your own community will show you many possibilities. Check with professional caregivers, the library, and your local AARP.

It is easier to share the care giving when there is a coordinator, but that person must be willing to hear all suggestions and discuss alternative options. Each person has to be honest and realistic about what they can and will do, so that there will be a reliable division of labor. As time goes by, responsibilities may change and expand. There will always be plenty to do at every level.

Remember people respond better when they are asked to do something rather than being told.

WHO CAN HELP?

Mother was very ill with cancer but despite constant offers of more help, my father assured us that he was holding up fine as the main caregiver. "I don't need help yet," he'd say. Then one day he walked down to his neighborhood bank and explained to the woman he usually dealt with there that he wanted to close one account and transfer funds to another. She listened carefully, then looked up at him and responded quietly, "Mr. Brown, you did that yesterday." Stunned, he walked home, picked up the phone and called me. "I think I do need some help," he admitted. From that day on, I began spending the nights with

Mother. Dad got some much-needed sleep; I was grateful for the opportunity to provide something that they both needed.

Ask and you shall receive!

Include the Family

Care giving is neither sexist nor age-limited — an equal opportunity service.

There is a great benefit for the elderly to be around young people, though high activity levels of very small children may be exhausting over a long period of time. Be aware of your elder's level of tolerance. Enlisting the help of your older children offers you a great opportunity to teach responsibility and thoughtfulness. Letting them choose from a variety of needed contribu-tions may make them feel more personally involved and in control. Allowing them the right to refuse sometimes will ease feelings of resentment. Keep in mind that children are also helping when they begin doing for themselves what you previously did for them.

Ask For Help

Most people are not good mind readers! Be specific in asking for and offering help. Friends and neighbors may be willing to help if you ask. Young adults may be interested in earning money doing special errands. Sources for back-up when you are unable to do your usual eldercaring will bring you peace of mind. Keep a list of these "angels" for emergencies.

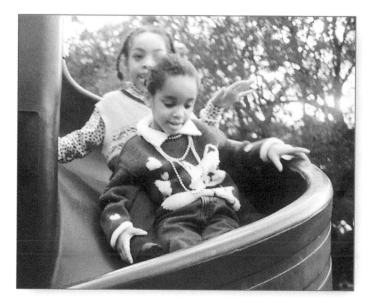

Be Creative

If you have a friend who is in the same boat, share some responsibilities. When you're visiting, can you stop by your

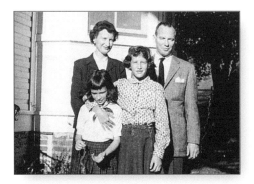

friend's relative, too? Go on outings together — then everybody has fun and you can giggle afterwards about the absurdities.

Consult Your Professionals

Professionals rely on calls to keep abreast of changes or problems. If possible, call during waking hours! Take advantage of help and information from local support groups.

In-Laws

Being an "in-law" involved with care giving may present different challenges. Ask your spouse for suggestions on how to help. Different kinds of emotional ties may make eldercaring easier for some and more difficult for others

Don't Be Critical

When working with others, avoid pointing a finger. Instead, focus on sending positive "I" messages and avoid hurt feelings. For example, instead of saying,

"You didn't do what you were supposed to," say "I wish we could coordinate our schedules better." The most important thing you can do for any relationship during shared eldercaring is to keep lines of communication open and your priorities in line.

"I believe that every human mind feels pleasure in doing good for another."

— Thomas Jefferson

How To Begin: Research Pays Off

Use the library, internet or bookstore to investigate organizations and ideas that can meet your special eldercaring needs.

Have a family conference

Plan a family meeting or conference call to assess problems, brainstorm options and keep everyone informed. Have an agenda, keep focused and take notes which can be circulated later. Plan follow-up meetings as needed. Give other caregivers the opportunity to blow off steam and release frustrations.

N o t e s

> *"Light is the task where many share the toil."*
>
> — Homer
>
> *"Hot heads and cold hearts never solved anything."*
>
> — Billy Graham

Make decisions together

Deal with other family members up front and honestly. Express your thoughts clearly and be willing to listen to theirs. If possible, *agree to agree!!* (Or else, you may end up doing it all yourself.)

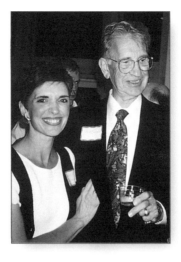

Divide up responsibilities

Decide among you who has what responsibilities — taxes, insurance, errands, outings, shopping, health care, meals and grooming.

My mother always gave us a little "sunshine" when we weren't feeling well. A "sunshine" was a gift of food, flowers or something fun. Give a little "sunshine" to anyone you know who is being cared for or is eldercaring.

All efforts are appreciated

Visiting in itself is a valuable contribution to care giving. Consider reading aloud — the newspaper or a short article will entertain both of you. If you are not the primary caregiver, visit, call and write regularly. A postcard can elevate spirits.

Don't ask someone to do a favor and then tell them how to do it. This will cause resentment and an unwillingness to help in the future. Allow them to be creative.

"Call it a clan, call it a network, call it a tribe, call it a family. Whatever you call it, whoever you are, you need one."
— Sarah Ban Breathnach,
Simple Abundance, A Daybook of Comfort and Joy,
(New York: Warner Books, 1995).

N o t e s

❤ TIPS FOR CAREGIVERS

❤ Keep current. A call a day keeps a crisis away!! It will also make you aware of subtle changes.

❤ Plan ahead. Make your plans known to fellow caregivers in time for them to make suitable arrangements in your absence. Not everyone works well under pressure or under time constraints.

❤ Write it down. Put a large block calendar by your elder's phone and have each of the caregivers record when they will be by and what activity they plan to do: a lunch outing, doctor's appointment, hair care, etc. This will keep your elder informed and help coordinate care giving efforts.

❤ Keep a visitors book. Use a notebook to record visits and leave messages for other caregivers.

❤ Say "thank you" often. Encourage all caregivers by acknowledging their efforts.

"If you can't excel with talent, triumph with effort."

— Dave Weinbaum

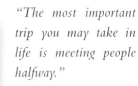

"The most important trip you may take in life is meeting people halfway."

— Henry Boye

"Service is the rent that we pay for our room on earth."

— Lord Halifax

YOUR RIGHTS

The Family and Medical Leave Act: Under this 1993 legislation, employees must be offered up to twelve weeks of unpaid leave to care for an ill family member. This applies to businesses with fifty or more employees and an employee who has been with the company for at least one year and accomplished 1,250 hours of work in the past twelve months.

Sharing Is Important Because . . .

Variety is the spice of life.
Caretaking can be lonely.
You can't do it all forever.
Many hands make light work.
The more people, the more.
ideas, the more solutions.

Notes

> "Shared laughter
> offers us pleasure
> during the fun times and
> a resilient strength dur-
> ing distress."
>
> — Carmen Renee Berry
> and Tamara Traeder,
> *Girlfriends: Invisible
> Bonds Enduring Ties*
> (Berkeley: Wildcat
> Canyon Press, 1995, p. 90)

TECHNOLOGY TO THE RESCUE

When Mother had to go into the hospital for surgery, I was the only one who could be with her. Knowing how difficult it is to place long distance calls from the hospital, I took my laptop computer with me. I could e-mail my brother and sisters to keep them apprised of Mother's status and, as she recovered, she enjoyed hearing their messages and passing along her own through me. It cheered her up immensely. Aren't computers a godsend!

Technology can play a positive caregiving role in more ways than one:

• Researching on the internet can make patients and caregivers feel more in control of decision making.

• For the physically challenged but mentally alert elder, learning to use a computer can add to self-esteem and even be a status symbol with contemporaries (and grandchildren!).

FOURTEEN FRIENDS' CAREGIVER'S CREED

I will do my best
for my loved-one.

I will be open to advice.

I will acknowledge
tensions, and find ways
to work around them.

I will share responsibilities
as well as credit.

I will remember the needs
of my own family.

I will remind myself that
I am not responsible for
everyone's happiness.

• Communication by e-mail is a "call" you can take when you feel up to it. In the meantime, it waits for you.

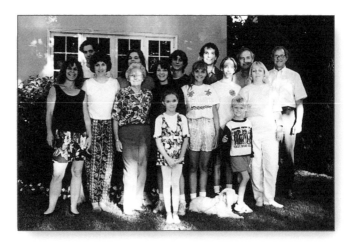

Notes

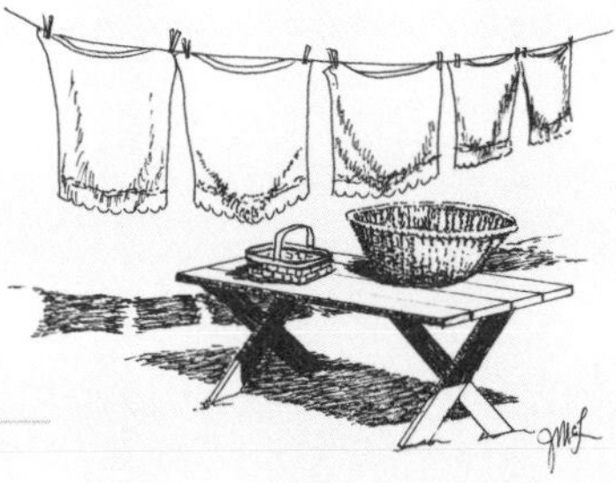

_____

_____

_____

_____

_____

_____

_____

_____

_____

_____

_____

_____

_____

_____

_____

_____

_____

_____

_____

_____

_____

_____

_____

_____

_____

_____

_____

Food was always an integral part of the relationship I had with my great aunt. Childless, she managed to spoil the children of her friends and family with her love of cooking. When visiting her you were asked to give a list of favorite foods. Lamb chops, artichokes with hollandaise sauce and fresh cabbage (not staples at my house!) were on my list. Today, my treasured memory of her request is a childhood photo of my communion day, holding her gift of a raw cabbage wrapped in white tissue paper, tied with a blue ribbon.

The Italians have an old saying, "There is no problem a little food won't solve." And who of us can't recall a time when our own troubles were temporarily forgotten, replaced by the aroma and taste of a favorite food? It should be of no surprise, then, that food and comfort appear inseparably linked. This relationship of "food/comfort" enhances good health with the delight of eating. My aunt knew that. She knew that far more than good health, food provided time for a family to be together, to talk and share and savor the day.

COMFORT FOOD AND NUTRITION

COMFORT FOOD

The pleasures of good food don't disappear with aging. For those in our care, it is important to identify their needs and wants regarding food choices. Involve them if possible in occasional meal planning by asking how they prepared family dishes. Simple nutritional alterations of their old favorite recipes can keep alive the pleasant memories of family gatherings long gone. Giving our loved ones special pleasures of favorite foods or beverages, though not on their recommended diets, can nourish their minds and souls far more than their bodies. Your efforts will make them feel special and loved. The comforting routine of anticipating an afternoon out for ice cream, a favorite slice of pie, or a good hot cup of coffee brings pleasure to eldercaring. And for the long distance caregivers there are many companies that deliver foods and beverages unique to the season and richly extravagant . . . ruby red grapefruit from Florida, chocolate chunk cookies, imported chocolates, and specialty coffees, to name just a few.

Eating is an affirmation of life: it is also a requirement for healthy living. Because the metabolism

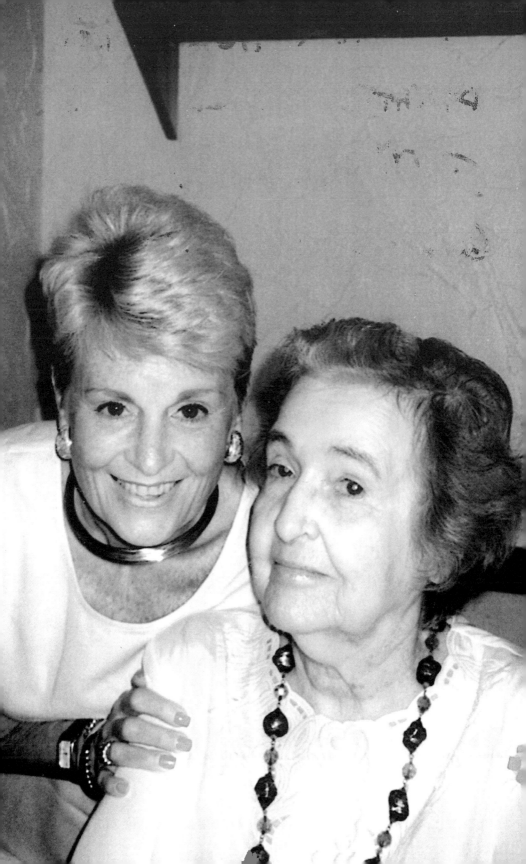

of an older person slows down, typically fewer calories are burned, and thus appetites decrease. These metabolic changes

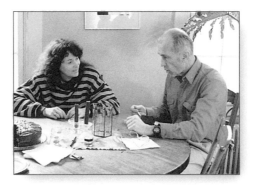

are a major problem that need the attention of the caregiver. As everyone knows, proper diet is essential to good health. To maintain a healthy diet, many types of vegetables, fruits, rice, and grains should be served daily. The rule of many nutritionists can be summarized by the following formula: low-fat/high-fiber; low-alcohol/high-fluid; low caffeine/ high vegetable/fruit. To make the best use of time, make mealtimes a special part of the day.

Enjoyment

Since Mother's stroke, she has residual aphasia (jumbled speech). An activity that doesn't require much conversation is cooking. Making cheese straws when she visits is familiar and fun for both of us. With help, she remembers what to do next. The dough isn't as smooth as it used to be and the straws aren't as straight, but who cares! She feels happy, useful and competent. And the cheese straws taste great!

Food and drink are a natural part of celebration. The twilight years provide a unique ambiance that runs the gamut from reminiscing to wonderfully wise and humorous insight for today's current events. So, gather those folks of vintage years, add a little music, and conversation, and bring on the food. Celebrate life!

Dining is an occasion, and fellowship at mealtime can make a regular meal an experience. Try to create some special times for your loved one — vary the menu, make meals surrounding a theme and try to add some fluff — decorate the table with a simple thing like adding festive napkins. Creating a memorable meal can make visits more exciting.

Epicureus had a great idea: "Eat, drink and be merry, for tomorrow you may die!"

Past Pleasures

Family holidays weren't complete without Smithfield ham and Mother's homemade biscuits. Before her stroke, she could make biscuits without a recipe and taught my daughter and me her technique.

Now she silently supervises my making her biscuits before family dinners. She's still the chef and I'm the sous chef.

Food memories and mouth-watering aromas — we all have our favorites. From the smell of cinnamon rolls cooking on Saturday mornings to that Thanksgiving turkey roasting in the oven — we constantly tap our memory bank when we experience euphoric recall. If our loved one no longer has the ability or inclination to make these favorites today, then we, as caregivers, certainly can be creative enough to try our hand at reproducing or finding a close substitute to celebrate old times.

> *"Give me sunshine —*
> *if not on my face,*
> *then . . . on my plate!"*
>
> — Margery Friedman
> "Menu for the Winter Blahs"
> (*The Washington Post*,
> February 25, 1998)

You'll be surprised at how elders are pleased that you appreciated their past efforts. It's pay-back time!!

Using old, familiar recipes (or healthier versions) can be a real hit!

My mom still makes cornstarch pudding that I remember watching my grandmother cook on a wood stove. Mom was delighted when I asked her to share the following recipe. It is taken from a 1926 cookbook published by "The Ladies of the Green Park Grange" in Green Park, Perry County, Pennsylvania.

Corn Starch Pudding

Beat 1 egg and 2 cups sugar, add 2 tablespoons cornstarch.
Stir in 1 pint boiling milk and 1 teaspoon butter.
Flavor with 1 teaspoon vanilla.
Cook over low heat until thickened. Pour into individual dessert dishes and cool. Refrigerate until serving.

If dining is difficult — simplify! Prepare easy-to-eat foods and set the table with only one utensil! Helping to sustain dignity may ultimately aid in digestion!

EAT FOR THE HEALTH OF IT!

My great-aunt lived in our home with my husband and me and our three sons from the time she was 95 until she was 102 years old. She weighed 90 pounds soaking wet but had a voracious appetite and some peculiar tastes. I miss catching her trying to take a few sips from the dill pickle jar. I'm glad I didn't scold her.

Eating healthily goes for all ages as the new buzzwords are "low-fat" and "low-cholesterol." This is exactly what nutritionists prescribe for the aging. Of course, proper vitamins, minerals, fiber and exercise are important, too.

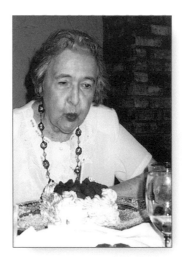

Older people eat less food mainly because they are less hungry. Although they need as many vitamins and minerals as they ever did, These must come from less total food intake. So, make every bite count. Take a close look at your elder's diet. Too little or too much of certain foods might explain increased depression or lack of energy and nervousness. Vigilance to medical needs and diets is important, plus eating smaller portions more times a day rather than three large meals will help sustain energy levels. Fluids are extremely important. Water intake should amount to one quart daily. Perhaps to make this fun, you can label a quart jar of water in the fridge as "Dad's Jet Fuel." This may create some whimsical conversation.

REMEMBER – "Running on a full tank will get you where you want to go!"

❤ Tips for Healthy Eating

❤ Key words are *variation* and *moderation*. A good diet includes different vegetables, fruits, rice, grains. An occasional doughnut is fine; a pound of carrots daily is not necessary.

❤ Throw out the salt shaker. Use salt substitutes and other spices.

❤ For fast food dining, avoid deluxes, doubles, whoppers, and so on. Instead order salads, grilled chicken or fish, chile, single burgers and thin crust pizza (toppings of green peppers, mushrooms and onions are terrific)!

❤ Alcohol — no more than 2 drinks per day.

❤ Restaurants — avoid butter, cream and cheese sauces, fatty meats (order lean cuts), fried foods and mayonnaise.

Notes

> "We can do no great
> things, only small
> things with great love."
> — Mother Teresa

LIKE AGING WINE . . . TASTES CHANGE

We are constantly changing. During the later stages of aging, change may be accelerated and seem more acute than ever before. My 82-year-old mother recently began to have periodic stomach cramps. Being aware of exactly when this occurred made her conscious of the fact that it was only when she ate chocolate. So-o-o she decided to test her hunch.

> *"There is no duty we so much underrated as the duty of being happy. By being happy we sow anonymous benefits upon the world."*
>
> — Robert Louis Stevenson

She waited a few days, then once again ate more chocolate. The cramps came back but she had solved the mystery. Somewhat a sad scenario for chocolate lovers; but with this same method she rid herself of frequent digestive problems which she figured out were caused by leafy greens in salads. Coffee, too, had to be cut from her diet.

❤ TIPS FOR DIET DIAGNOSIS

❤ Watch out for rich, spicy foods.

❤ Keep a journal of meals that are digestively unfriendly.

❤ Foods can affect moods. Too many sweets may bring on a depressed and/or tired feeling — take a feelings pulse after meals!

❤ It's never too late to try new foods — variety is the spice of life! Just be aware of their effect.

HINTS FOR HELPERS

• Microwaves are simple to operate and make food preparation quick and easy — a great investment for someone living alone.

• Help create a shopping list. A pre-visit call to pick up items before you arrive may save time and keep the pantry stocked for a rainy day!

• Let them eat cake . . . it's nutritious **enough!**

Mother needs the calories . . . I take her to the bakery and let her pick out an eclair for dinner (she loves them) and a pastry for the next morning.

TAKE TIME TO SMELL THE HERBS!

My dad wanted to do all the cooking when he visited so that our meal would be ready when my husband amd I got home from work. It was amazing that he could take perfectly good ingredients and turn them into inedible, unrecognizable food. He was determined to improve, however. One day, wanting to acknowledge the effort he was making, we complimented him on his "spaghetti sauce." When we returned from running errands that day, we discovered that he had cooked another gallon of it! On another occasion, we

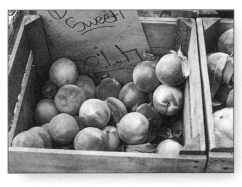

returned home to discover the counters covered with Key Lime pies — an effort to improve the meringue. This search for perfection was a source of many surprises and many a good laugh!

There is considerable focus these days on food and beverages that provide not only nutritional value but medicinal value as well. Interestingly, the field of psychiatry is currently researching aromatherapy as possible treatment for some forms of mental illness. Herbal principles are used in many modern

Notes

_____
_____
_____
_____
_____
_____
_____
_____
_____
_____
_____

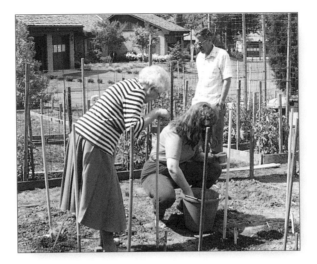

medications. Caffeine in coffee, tea, cola and cocoa is used in medications for the treatment of migraine headaches due to its effect on blood vessels. Theophylline, a chemical cousin of caffeine, commonly found in tea, is used in asthma medications. Theobromine, a chemical in cocoa, acts as a heart stimulant and a diuretic in some modern medicines. Ginger is used to control gastrointestinal disorders and is a common ingredient found in soft drinks. Cinnamon and peppermint oils, mustard seed, and cloves are all used in scientifically prepared medicines, although most of us are more familiar with their use in foods, teas, and candies.

"HERE'S TO YOU!"

My friend and his wife meet every Thursday evening at the retirement home where his mother has an apartment to have a drink with her. Occasionally, they stay for dinner or take her out, but more often the cocktail hour is what they spend together, a time that fits into their busy schedules and gives her an occasion to anticipate. If alcohol is not included in the diet of your loved one, substitute a soda. The point is the occasion, not the beverage. Once in awhile, take an hors d'oeuvre. Recreate in their current circumstance the festive tradition of sharing the day over a drink.

Mini refrigerators and microwave ovens are great, not only for college students, but also for residents of assisted living facilities. They eat meals in a communal dining room and do not have their own kitchens, but having the ability to keep a supply of some of their favorite treats, hot or cold, makes life more fun and better tasting.

N o t e s

For many of us, our parents, especially our mothers, have a natural talent for causing us to feel guilty. "Why don't you ever call me?" is a familiar refrain. My mother has taken this one step further . . . when she calls me and I'm not home, she refuses to leave a message on my answering machine. Consequently, I never know when she has tried to reach me. Eventually, when I call her, she says in an accusing tone of voice, "I called you. Why weren't you there?" The first time this happened, I actually found myself feeling guilty. Then I realized how ludicrous this was and was able to laugh at the situation. Unfortunately, it is not always this easy to recognize and put an end to unnecessary guilt feelings.

COMMON FEELINGS OF GUILT

Feelings of guilt are very common when you are involved in eldercaring. These feelings can be self-inflicted or can be imposed on us by other people. When the guilt is legitimate, it spurs us to do better. When it is unwarranted, it only causes anxiety and hampers our ability to make sound decisions and to give quality care.

Self-inflicted guilt often results from the anger and the resentment we feel towards the elder. Anger

GUILT

occurs when our new role as caregiver radically changes our daily routines. Demands on our time and restraints on our freedom lead to feelings of resentment. It is annoying to be required to give up our limited free time, and it is distressing when eldercaring interferes with career or family time. Yet we may simultaneously feel that we can never do enough as the caregiver, and that we are not able to handle the situation well. When we observe pain and sorrow in an elder's life, it causes uncomfortable feelings and a desire to "fix" everything. Realistically we know that this is not possible. We cannot solve their every problem or provide their missing happiness. These conflicting emotions lead to guilt which can be a constant companion for the caregiver.

Guilt may also be imposed on us by outside sources. Chastisement can come from the elder, from other caregivers, or even from a friend. For instance, we may feel guilty when the elder expresses displeasure over the brevity of our visits. In this case, we should ask ourselves whether staying longer would truly prevent the unhappiness or just delay it. It is not uncommon for fellow caregivers

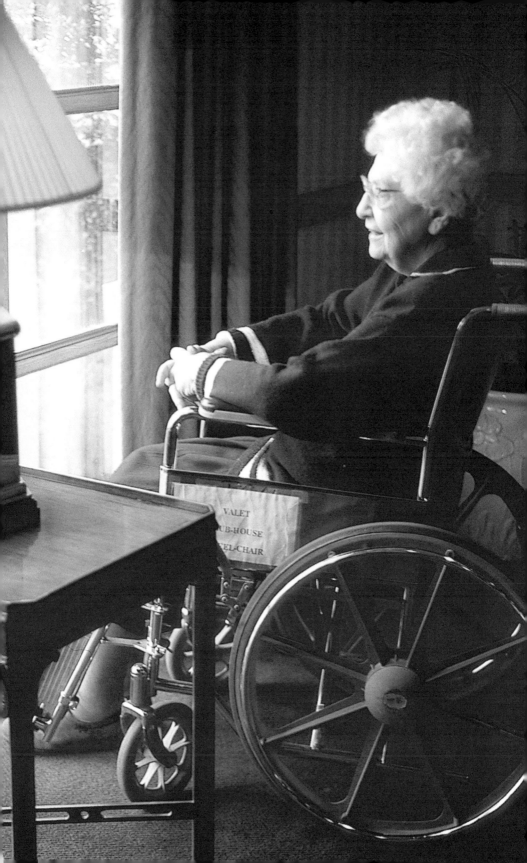

to feel that they are bearing more than their share of the responsibility, and their comments may cause feelings of guilt.

Having a conscience sets up the probability of occasional feelings of guilt. We must be able to distinguish between useful and legitimate guilt as opposed to guilt that is harmful and undeserved. The former can motivate us to get things done while the latter only serves to dishearten us. Curtailing our feelings of guilt can renew the energy we need for effective care giving. Recognize and be proud of what you are giving and give generously.

To determine if the guilt you are feeling is warranted, ask yourself if you have done everything that is practical and necessary within your own parameters. Will doing more significantly help a given situation or not? Bear in mind, what is important is ensuring the quality of care and meeting the realistic needs of the elderly. Quiet the guilt.

GUILTY OR NOT GUILTY?

Make a list of things that make you feel guilty. Examine the underlying reasons and determine if a solution is within your power. Consider that your elder may feel guilty because they are imposing on you, while you are feeling guilty that you don't have time to do more. Inducing guilt may also be a control tactic. Recognize it for what it is.

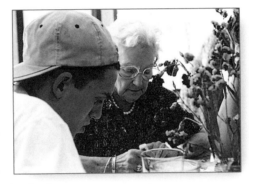

Common causes of guilt feelings include:

• You don't have the usual amount of time to spend with your children and spouse.

• You don't have enough time to help your elder.

• You don't have enough time to do your job as well as before.

• You don't have enough time to care for yourself such as exercising and preparing nourishing meals.

• You don't feel you have the skills necessary to do a good job of eldercaring.

• You have negative feelings towards fellow family caregivers.

• You feel resentment towards your elders because of the demands they place on you physically and emotionally.

MANAGING GUILT

It is hard to think clearly when you are under a lot of pressure or stress so consider letting an outsider help you focus on whether your guilt is realistic and help you find ways to come to terms with it. Counselors, pastors, your spouse, friends, and support groups can all be sources of help and comfort.

"Action and care will in time wear down the strongest frame, but guilt and melancholy are poisons of quick dispatch."

— Thomas Paine

Even though my mother-in-law has an aversion to leaving messages on my machine, I now know that she has called by checking my caller ID.

Notes

> *"A lot of guilt comes from the feeling that we have more influence than we really do."*
>
> — Harold Kushner,
> *How Good Do We Have to Be? A New Understanding of Guilt and Forgiveness*
> (Boston: Little, Brown and Company, 1996, p. 58)

At all costs I avoid regret. Shortly after Dad died I felt guilty about the times I was feeling angry over his confusion, and feeling fed up about the constant care. Then I consciously thought and talked about how much I gave Dad . . . the days of worry, the calls, the care, the unending love and support and time. I only resolved to feel proud. I have no regrets.

YES, YOU ARE GOING TO FEEL GUILTY!

Some things you can do to manage these feelings are:

• Remember that no one can make you feel guilty unless you allow it.

• Remember that experts were beginners.

• Don't let conflicts from the past cause guilt in the present.

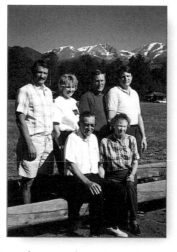

• Don't put off things that need to be done. Procrastination can cause feelings of guilt to grow.

• Concentrate on what can be done today and in the future. Anguishing over what you should have done will not solve anything.

• Remind yourself that "what other people think of me is none of my business!"

ALL YOU CAN DO IS YOUR BEST!

"Please don't leave . . ." is a statement my mother often made after our visit. I now realize that the guilt it caused could have been avoided if I had timed my visit so that my departure would coincide with one of her activities or a meal.

Volunteer in your community as a way of thanking others who are kind to your loved ones. This is particularly rewarding if your own elders live far away and you are unable to do all you would like for them. The old adage that "what goes around, comes around" applies here. Try volunteering at your church, Meals on Wheels, nursing homes or hospice. Caring for, encouraging and visiting other elders can also be therapeutic when the responsibility of caring for your own elders has ended. Turn regrets into positive action.

"Please do not feel personally, irrevocably responsible for everything. That's my job! Love, God."

— Meiji Stewart, *Keep Coming Back* (Del Mar, CA: Puddle Dancer Press, p. 128).

> *"Concern should drive us into action and not into depression."*
>
> — Karen Horney
> *Simple Abundance,*
> *A Daybook of Comfort*
> *and Joy* by Sarah
> Ban Breathnach
> (New York: Warner
> Books, 1995)

When my mother pouts and says, "Where have you been, I haven't seen you . . ." I have adopted a new strategy to alleviate my guilt. I turn the conversation around and tell her what a great time I had with my husband just like she and Daddy used to have together. Getting her to remember old times makes her enjoy hearing about the times we're enjoying now.

THE TIME HAS COME

Avoid "blanket" promises like "I'll never put you in a nursing home" or "I won't let you die alone." They can haunt you as the situation changes.

Deciding the timing and whether or not to withhold extraordinary medical measures when treating a terminally ill parent can cause guilt even when it has been agreed upon beforehand. An adult

Notes

it was fun and fairly easy to manage; but they were isolated from people their own age, and I was anxious and guilty about my own time. Moving them into a retirement community was the right decision. I don't have any guilt about what was best for all of us.

❤ TIPS FOR CAREGIVERS

❤ Express your feelings to your loved one now. If you aren't ready to express love in general, pick out a few instances you were appreciative of and talk about those.

❤ Record family stories or special memories.

❤ Record the names of family members in old photographs. Can other relatives help identify old photographs that you may find later? Don't wait to ask!

❤ Get information needed to trace genealogy — even though you may not be interested, your children or future generations may be.

❤ Record history of special belongings that will be inherited by family members. They will be more meaningful and appreciated.

❤ Encourage grandchildren to interact more and build memories of their grandparents. They will be thankful; if not now, later.

❤ Trying to make up for a lifetime of regrets is impossible.

child or family member may even wonder if his motives are completely pure. The assistance of a medical professional can alleviate some of this anxiety. They can clarify the consequences of your actions such as letting you know what responsibility the doctors will have to take when a patient is hospitalized at a certain stage of their illness.

KNOW YOUR OWN LIMITATIONS

I know my limitations as a person. I knew what I could do for my parents and what I could not do. They lived with me for five years. At the beginning

Notes

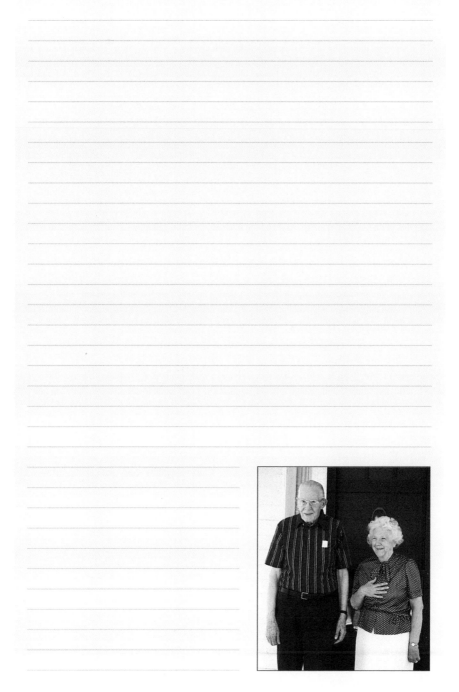

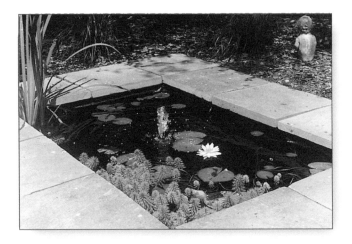

"But memory is what ultimately gives us power over death, by keeping the person alive in our hearts. Memory is what gives us power over time, by keeping the past present so that it cannot fade and rob us of what we once held precious."

— Harold Kushner, *How Good Do We Have to Be? A New Understanding of Guilt and Forgiveness* (Boston: Little, Brown and Company, 1996, p. 164)

"GUILT IS A FOUR LETTER WORD," is a sentence packed with meaning. You don't need a dictionary definition of guilt. You know it when you feel it. It isn't shame, contrition, penitence or remorse; it's guilt. Guilt, not meaning "I robbed the bank," but guilt meaning, "I could have done better or more."

So when does "guilt" become a four letter word, an expletive that your mother taught you not to use?

Guilt becomes a four letter word when it is used to manipulate others. When your mother begins a phone conversation with a sigh and, "Oh, you never come to see me," you feel guilty, and, on the way over to visit her, manipulated. Guilt has become a four letter word.

"You never call," I say with a sigh at the beginning of the conversation with my first born now residing in the far away Midwest. And then I hear myself sounding like my mother. Well, perhaps Mother's message is not intended to create guilt but is, instead, an expression of love!

"Things do not change; we change."

— Henry David Thoreau

"Just because someone throws you the ball, you don't have to catch it."

— Richard Carlson, PhD, *Don't Sweat the Small Stuff* (New York: Hyperion, 1997)

N o t e s

My friend helps maintain quality of life as an octogenarian by swimming five days a week at the local recreation center. She lives with a daughter who drops her off at the pool on the way to work. When the routine began seven years ago, she was able to walk home after exercising. Although her physical and mental powers have declined somewhat, she has made many friends at the community center who make sure she has a ride home every morning and see that she is safely into her house. The exercise continues to be good for her physically and the socialization with a wide age group keeps her mind active. She has become an inspiration to the women who know her, from the teenagers on the swim team to the middle-aged women who hope to be as active when they reach her age.

"Well people are disappearing. I should have known it was coming when the invalids became extinct. (Invalids disappeared shortly after the advent of Medicare, which demanded specific diagnostic labels even though none existed.)"

— Clifton K. Meador
(*New England Journal of Medicine*, February 10, 1994)

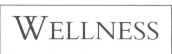

WELLNESS

The search for wellness seems to have become an obsession of this decade. The harder people work at it, the more impossible it is to attain. Medical science finds more disease than it can cure. Technological advances, such as MRI scanning, generate new terms, such as "unidentified bright objects" to refer to spots deep in the brain of uncertain significance. This is one more thing to worry about!

We grew up with the idea of the check-up, immunizations, and PAP smears. So what do the experts currently think we should do to stay well? Here is a collection of recommendations from three expert panels: Canadian Task Force on the Periodic Health Examination, U.S. Preventive Services Task Force, and the American College of Physicians. These policies are for adults whose history indicates no risk factors for disease (other than getting older!).

"How we lived five years ago has a lot to do with how healthy we are today. How we live today has a lot to do with how healthy we will be in five years. Or, in other words, 'The yoo-hoo you yoo-hoo into the forest is the yoo-hoo you get back.'" — Anonymous

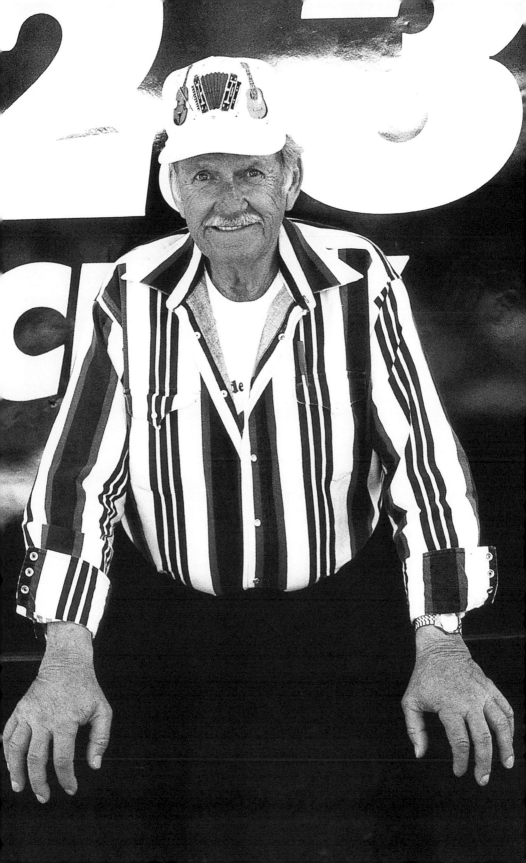

HEALTH TIPS

• Blood pressure measurement should be taken at every medical visit, and at least every two years.

• Breast examination by a physician should be performed annually for women over the age of 40. Breast palpation accounts for 50-67 percent of the value of breast exam and mammography.

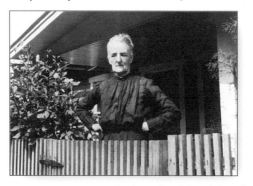

• Serum cholesterol should be measured every five years, starting in early adulthood.

• Mammography should be done annually, beginning at age 50 in all women, and every one to two years starting at the age of 35-40 years for women who have immediate family members with breast cancer. Some organizations recommend it annually for all women beginning at age 40.

• PAP smears should be taken every one to three years for sexually active women, starting at the age of first intercourse. If regular screening has yielded normal results, it is no longer necessary after age 65.

• Annual influenza vaccination should be given to people over age 65 with a pneumoccal vaccination once after age 65.

• Screening for colon cancer definitely should be done in those at high risk due to ulcerative colitis, polyps, familial polyposis, or those having immediate family with colon cancer. Annual screening for blood in the stool is effective but may miss two thirds of the tumors.

• Prostate cancer is the second leading cause of cancer deaths among men in the U.S. The American Cancer Society recommends that testing for prostate specific antigen (PSA) and digital rectal examination (DRE) be offered to men annually, beginning at age 50 and to younger men who are at high risk because of family history of the disease.

• For women at high risk of coronary artery disease, the American College of Physicians recomends estrogen and progesterone therapy (or estrogen alone for women who have had a hysterectomy). The routine use of hormone replacement in all post-menopausal women is controversial.

PROVIDE A SAFE ENVIRONMENT

Even small changes to the home place may go a long way to establishing a safer living space:

• Consider adding night lights in bathrooms, hallways and kitchen.

• Add grab bars and a stool to the shower or bathtub.

• Install a raised toilet seat with grab bars.

• Move furniture which may be in the way, make sure there is good lighting, eliminate clutter, and remove throw rugs which may lead to tripping.

• Check the thermostat on the hot water heater to minimize the danger of burns from overly heated bath water.

• Visit the various medical/handicap supply stores in your area to get other ideas to help provide a safer environment.

Everyday activities can be dangerous

Getting in and out of the bathtub or shower, using the stove or oven, using sharp tools or kitchen equipment, and driving when eyesight and reflexes begin to fail become dangerous activities.

Some safety precautions to consider:

• Install grab bars in bathrooms.

• Install handrails on steps and stairs indoors and outdoors.

• Have an electrician install a safety switch to shut off the stove at night.

• Attach bells to doors to alert the caregiver of night walking.

Maintain a comfortable body temperature

Try silk long underwear and layering clothes before turning the heat up excessively.

Notes

"Sometimes even music cannot substitute for tears."

— Paul Simon

It Takes More Than An Apple A Day

Make exercise a part of visits or daily activity as often as possible.

The President's Council on Physical Fitness and Sports has reported that much of the physical frailty attributed to aging is due to inactivity. Research confirms that exercise is important in the prevention and the treatment of heart disease, osteoporosis, diabetes, obesity and depression. Walking is a great exercise for just about everyone including elders, and often is a substitute for other meaningful activities or forms of exercise that they can no longer enjoy.

Get involved with your parent's health care provider

Bring along a list of questions to the doctor's office. Be assertive in getting the information you need. Don't leave until you have the answers.

Notes

The Key to Better Eating

Perhaps the key to better eating lies not only with the mechanics of preparing food but also with the social aspects of eating. Meal times should be social occasions spent eating in the company of others.

A recent study in which fifteen medical experts reviewed 4,500 studies on cancer and nutrition concluded that between 30 percent to 40 percent of all cancers could be prevented if people would simply change their eating habits and lifestyles.

Years ago the idea was that cancer was caused by bad things in our food supply. This new research concludes that cancer comes from not getting enough of the good things, reports Dr. Walter Willett of the Harvard School of Public Health, in a World Cancer Research Fund publication published by the American Institute for Cancer Research.

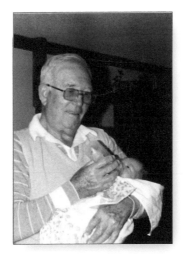

"Time spent with an elderly loved one pointing out what value they have been to us can do wonders. We can tell them how proud we are to be a part of their lives. We can tell them they are needed."

— Doug Manning,
When Love Gets Tough
(New York: Harper & Row, 1983, p. 89)

Driving

The need for help doesn't always coincide with insight into a difficulty. My dad called to request a loan to purchase a new car. He explained that his previous car was disabled when he fainted as he drove towards his cabin. He had crashed the car into his living room where it now occupied half of the living space. He was so oblivious of the situation that he thought he could continue living in the cabin and was focusing solely on the need for a new car. His insight into the ramifications of the situation was clearly impaired.

"No, Dad, you can't have the car tonight — or ever."

Has the time come to take away the car keys? It is important for the safety of the older person but also for the safety of other drivers!

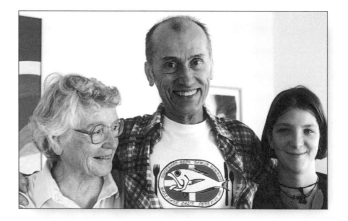

Most states have no laws tying the failure of cognitive abilities to driver's license renewal or suspension, so it's dependent on family members, caregivers, counselors and physicians to openly talk. To avoid conflict, anger and stress, Dr. Gray advises "slickness" over pure honesty. With dementia you can't appeal to the logic of the person because logic is increasingly unavailable.

"When we drive, especially familiar routes, our motor-habit memory takes over through repetition, repetition, repetition. That's what drives the car long after the person behind the wheel shouldn't be driving. At least, it works until they get into novel settings like ambulance sirens behind them or construction that necessitates a detour."

— Dr. Kevin Gray, Director
of Memory Disorders Clinic
of Dallas (*Ft. Worth Star Telegram*,
January 15, 1998)

"The idea of giving up driving should be presented as a medical prescription from the doctor rather than as informal advice from the family. This can be especially effective if your dad believes that the doctor's come to this conclusion after a thoughtful evaluation."

— Mark S. Lachs, M.D. ,
"Caring for Mom and Dad,"
(*Prevention*, January, 1998, p. 144)

Long before driving skills become impaired, consider enrollment in any of the many fine driving courses offered for older drivers. The American Automobile Association, AARP and the National Safety Council all offer courses specifically designed to improve and refresh the driving skills of older Americans. Call AAA about "Safe Driving for Mature Operators," AARP for "55 Alive/Mature Driving" or your local Chamber of Commerce for the National Safety

Notes

> "Humor is the great
> thing, the saving thing.
> The minute it crops up,
> all our irritations and
> resentments slip away,
> and a sunny spirit
> takes their place."
>
> — Mark Twain

Council courses offered near you. The Association of Driver Educators for the Disabled, P.O. Box 49, Edgerton, WI 53531, 608-884-8833 can give assistance in locating training programs for impaired drivers.

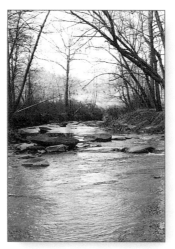

"If you're treading water, you're losing ground."

— Stephen W. Comisky

HYGIENE

Wash your hands!!

Infection Control Secret: Old fashioned hand washing! Numerous studies in professional journals are blaming epidemic outbreaks of bacterial and viral illness in hospitals, nursing homes, and child-care centers on the lack of hand washing. Donald Goldmann, a Boston epidemiologist, reports that the more short-handed or harried the staff, the more likely it is that they've forgotten to wash their hands. Don't worry about speaking up and possibly offending your health-care providers, he advises.

—"Wellness Matters," Lincoln National Life Insurance Co., Vol. XVIII, February 1998, p. 1.

Simplify personal hygiene

Bathing, brushing teeth, and other grooming and hygiene activities are often forgotten or overlooked as the elderly become more dependent. Some suggestions include:

• Add humor to bathing, like "We've got a hot date to get ready for."

• Substitute a sponge bath. It may be less threatening and is healthier for dry skin.

• Respect privacy, use a towel or robe to cover until the last minute.

• Put hygiene items out one at a time so as not to add to confusion. Get out toothbrush and toothpaste and accomplish that task alone. Put those items away before moving on to face washing, shaving, etc.

• Don't expect a perfect job.

"The highest reward for a man's toil is not what he gets for it, but what he becomes by it."

— John Ruskin

Notes

Like most of us, my work-a-day world falls week after week into a routine of schedules, appointments and commitments. However, this day was far from routine. The call came as I was completing a counseling session. My mother had been living independently in an assisted care facility in California. The residential manager explained that my mother had been drinking heavily since her roommate's stroke. They had been inseparable. When her roommate was moved to another facility, it was a tremendous loss for my mother. There was great concern for Mother's safety because the facility had no authority to keep her from leaving. I quickly made arrangements to fly to California, but when I arrived she was missing. After a prolonged search that day, the police returned her. She was found wandering seven miles from where she lived, confused, disoriented and intoxicated. I knew then that my mother had spent her last day living independently.

Today, for her safety, my mother resides in a secure facility about ten minutes from my home. She is doing quite well. So, for the present time, I can relax. Of my brothers and sisters, I am geographically situated the closest, so often my schedules, appointments and commitments must be put on hold and rearranged when mother needs my help. Juggling and rearranging my life are essential for my mother's care. Eldercaring is unpredictable.

ROLL WITH THE PUNCHES

The ability to be flexible in order to properly support a loved one, is a key element in eldercaring. For many of us the ability to "roll with the punches" becomes the name of the game. It is a skill that will help you handle the unexpected with less stress and anger. This flexibility, though often difficult and unwanted, can be cultivated over time. With patience, flexibility allows us to cope with the inevitable interruptions in their lives . . . and ours.

These interruptions in our adult lives are reminiscent of those experienced so frequently by our parents when they were raising us. Years ago, did our moms ever show anger when we forgot our lunch or books or assignments and called for their help? Probably! Would we have had a better day if Mom had accepted the fact that this oversight was just a "kid" thing? For sure! Would those loved ones in our care have a better

BE FLEXIBLE, BE PREPARED

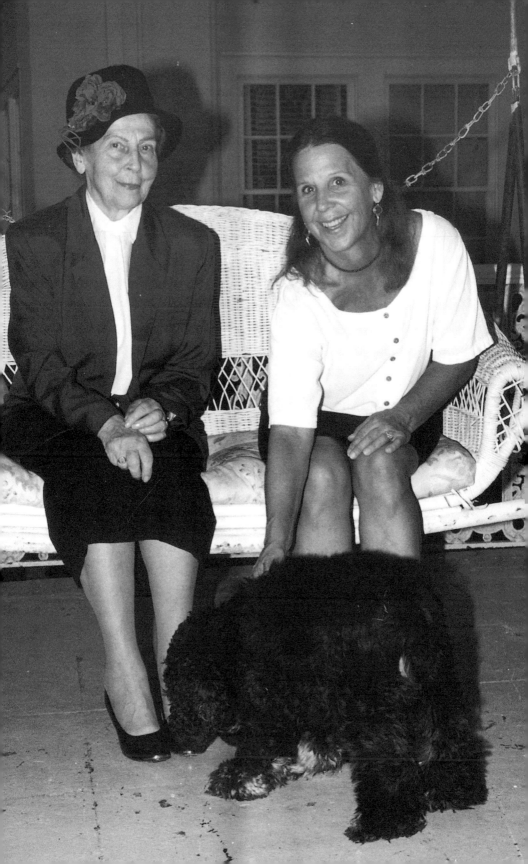

day if we accepted their oversights and interruptions as just an "elder" thing? Without a doubt! For their happiness, and our own, flexibility needs to become a part of our daily lives. Is this difficult? You bet it is! Is it going to get better? Most likely not, since aging happens to be irreversible.

Being flexible doesn't mean that our own lives have to be put on

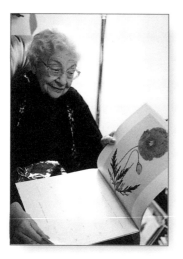

hold. Work schedules, social gatherings, other family activities, and private time can and should continue to flourish. After all, our parents lived their lives and managed to raise us at the same time. We can manage to care for our parents and raise our own lives to a higher level of satisfaction as well.

The secret, if it can be called that, is accepting the inevitable changes and remaining forever . . . flexible.

> *Flexibility is the antidote for rigidity.*

To keep a molehill from becoming a mountain overnight, be prepared for the unexpected. Are you prepared to find:

- Social security numbers (cards)
- Bank accounts and their numbers
- Safe deposit box and keys
- Names of doctors and phone numbers
- List of medications
- Health coverage information and cards
- House-related information: mortgage, insurance, utilities, etc.
- House and car keys
- Original copy of a will
- Birth certificate (exact place and date of birth)
- Marriage certificate
- Military discharge papers
- Citizenship papers.

It's like having children all over again — and you may not have nine months to get ready!

"Everyone wishes they'd known everything sooner!"

> — Nelson Demille,
> *The Talbot Odyssey*

> Use the sample forms in this journal to keep a record of significant information as well as personal and health developments. Project future needs and be ready to put a plan in place. Plan for different contingencies such as sudden total or partial dependence or supplemental care. Consult our chapter on "Sources for Help" for a list of associations, agencies and foundations that can provide information and publications. Add to our list with suggestions of your own.

"No day in which you learn something is a complete loss."

— David Eddings

BE PREPARED
AND START READING!

Eldercaring advice is available in magazines, newspapers and books and over the internet. Try using key words "care giving" to begin your search. Since you may have to jump in and make decisions from day one, have a plan for taking care of your personal responsibilities if it becomes necessary.

Frank discussion with your elder about what will need to be done in the future will help you be prepared. The roles are changing and you want your elders to be in control as long as possible and have a voice in their future. You need to know what arrangements they have made for themselves.

ARE YOU PREPARED FOR EMERGENCIES?

Make several index cards with information needed in emergencies. NOW!! They should include:

- Full name
- Address
- Phone number
- Primary doctor, name, address and phone number
- Medical insurance carrier with copy of front and back of I.D. card
- Allergies — especially medicines
- Medicines currently taken
- Any permanent disability or condition
- Person to notify in emergency
- Social Security number.

This is valuable information! Protect it as you would a credit card.

> *"We are all pilgrims on the same journey but some pilgrims have better road maps."*
>
> — Nelson DeMille,
> *The Talbot Odyssey*
> (New York:
> Delacorte, 1997)

ARE YOU PREPARED LEGALLY?

You need to find out if your elder has the following. Do they need updating? Are they necessary?

- Power of Attorney: Insures the continued handling of financial matters. Consider appointing more than one power of attorney or sequential powers of attorney.
- Living will and/or durable medical power of attorney: makes clear your elder's wishes regarding medical procedures if they are unable to make their wishes known.
- Guardian: an advocate for the elder.
- Up-to-date will: one that meets current legal requirements. Who is the executor? Consult an attorney.
- Access to documents: A safety deposit box is not the best place to keep the original of a will unless someone other than your elder has access. You only have access to a safety deposit box if your name is on the lease agreement. Without the key you will have to pay to have the box drilled.

"A little bit added to what you've already got gives you a little bit more."

— P. G. Wodehouse

Notes

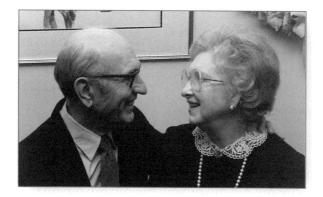

ARE YOU PREPARED FINANCIALLY?

I wanted to run a few last errands for my parents before I left for the airport. We went to the bank to make a deposit, and as I presented the items to be deposited I asked for the balance on the account. To my surprise, the young teller said the account had been closed. She related that my mother and father had come in last week and demanded that the account be closed and a new one established. Mom looked at the teller dumbfounded, and said she had done no such thing! The manager came over to confirm that, yes, the account had been closed. Mother was indignant and insisted she didn't remember any of this!

The many electronic fund transfers which deposited their annuities, retirement checks and social security monies, as well as paid all their recurring bills, were suspended and were probably now in cyberspace. The bank manager explained, as I was seething with anger, that it was impossible to reestablish the old account or transfer the EFT's to the newly established account and denied that they had any responsibility to contact me or my brother who were co-signers on the old account.

DO YOU KNOW?

• What are current sources of income? Social Security? Pensions? Interest? Dividends? Will pensions continue for surviving spouse?

• Are there sufficient financial assets? Make plans for assistance if needed.

• Have you arranged for joint bank accounts or to become a co-signer? Use direct deposit. Will the bank call you if your parent tries to close the account without your knowledge?

• Is there a financial planner/ accountant?

• Is there a stockbroker? Does the broker hold the stock certificates? If not, where are they? How is the stock held (individually, jointly)?

Notes

> *"Nothing in life is to be feared. It is only to be understood."*
>
> — Marie Curie

• Do you know the difference between Medicaid and Medicare? Is there supplemental insurance (Medigap insurance)? Is there additional insurance for dental, prescriptions, nursing home and long term care? Where are the policies, I.D. cards and phone numbers for contacts?

• Are there tangible assets (silver coins, for instance) in a box under the bed? Those who lived through the Depression often have valuables tucked away for the return of bad times. Yes, sometimes spouses do keep assets like cash hidden from each other.

• Is there life insurance? Who is the beneficiary? Make sure that this is up to date.

• Are there survivor benefits from employers such as additional employer paid life insurance?

"Procrastination is like a credit card — it's a lot of fun 'til you get the bill!"

— Christopher Parker

ARE YOU PREPARED MEDICALLY?

Beginning a dialogue with your elder's physician will help in later decision-making and care.

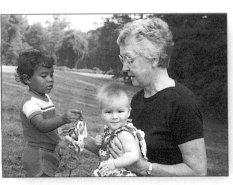

• Who is the primary care doctor? Where is the office? What is the phone number? Which hospital do you go to for emergencies?

• Are there any specialists involved in regular care? Who is the dentist? Podiatrist? Optician? Audiologist?

• What medications are taken regularly? What are they for? Are they all consolidated at one pharmacy? Where? How often can/should they be refilled? The weekly pill boxes with four compartments for each day are a great help when keeping track of multiple medications. Get two and be prepared for two weeks. Find out which pharmacies deliver.

• Have you consulted a geriatric psychiatrist? Depression, substance abuse and over-medication are common problems causing psychological distress in the elderly.

• Can you find the eyeglass prescription?

N o t e s

> "There are only
> two ways to live your
> life. One is as though
> nothing is a miracle.
> The other is as though
> everything is a miracle."
>
> — Albert Einstein

The phone rang, and even though she doesn't drive anymore I heard my mother say, "You have taken my car keys!" Thirty seconds ago we had just hung up having had the same conversation. Shortly, the phone would ring again, and Mother would ask for her keys. Had she forgotten she called? Was it the keys? Did she need attention? What did she need? We later learned Mother's behavior was symptomatic of Alzheimer's and she couldn't help herself. We dealt with it by hiding extra sets of random keys. Now, whenever Mother calls, I can tell her to try looking in one of several places where I have hidden sets of keys. Mother has the comfort of finding the "missing/stolen keys." She feels in control; I feel less frustrated.

FRUSTRATION

Frustration is experienced in almost every aspect of eldercaring. Many of the frustrations arise from situations which involve the following:

• Dealing with behaviors, habits, and attitudes of the elderly.

• Meeting the elder's physical needs and emotional demands.

• Having unrealistic expectations of the elderly.

Frustration causes feelings of discouragement, confusion, disappointment and anger. Looking at the causes of frustration and learning to understand and handle frustrating situations will help caregivers to feel better. When you feel better, satisfactory solutions are easier to find.

Traits and attitudes commonly associated with the elderly are frequently annoying. Repeating the same story over and over or not remembering what to do next and why is extremely irritating. Feelings of irritation may stem from a fear of developing these traits ourselves. These are normal feelings. Caregivers become annoyed and impatient when under stress or in a hurry themselves. Consequently, little problems become big ones. Understanding that frustrations are inherent in eldercaring is important.

Effectively dealing with them is a big step further. Begin by finding ways to relieve tension. For instance, bring humor into the situation and have a good laugh. Laughter is great! *When asked if Alzheimer's runs in my family, I answer, I don't remember!* Seeing the humorous side can untie the knots of irritation.

A change of atmosphere or scenery works wonders for dispelling tension. "I'm going for a walk with my headset," is my escape

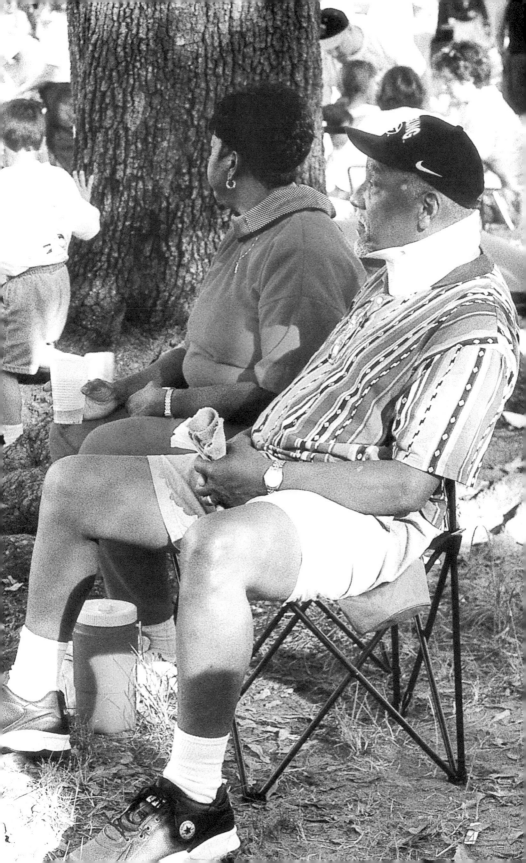

statement. Identify and eliminate stressful parts of activities. "If that's what she wants to wear, what difference does it make if it doesn't match?" If you find yourself falling into the same uncomfortable or annoying rut, change your pattern. Plan visits for a different time or place. Dementia breeds anger and feeds on itself. Back off and cool down. Take a few breaths, stretch your muscles, yell into a pillow, talk with a friend. Consider this as a new motto: Slow down, simplify, and be sensitive. Embrace the moments that are good . . . savor them and make note of them to remember later.

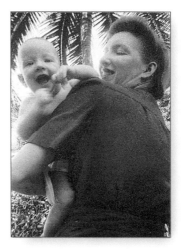

Empathy and patience remain important. Try to relate to feelings of helplessness, fear, and isolation, and try to understand that these feelings may be the result of stubbornness or the need for attention. Find simple ways of helping everyone reduce frustration. When you have a happy visit or a genuine moment of closeness, write about it in this journal to read again during the tough times.

It is helpful to examine personal expectations and to determine whether they are realistic or necessary. Unrealistic expectations for the elderly by the caregiver cause frustration. Adjust your expectations — not just the grand but the modest — for each visit, gathering, and time of family togetherness. With reasonable expectations, it will be easier to exceed them and feel satisfaction and pleasure.

Keep in mind that frustration is a normal emotion. Realize you are only human and are trying your best. Some frustration is unavoidable.

SOMETIMES I WANT TO STOMP MY FEET AND SCREAM!

Always feisty, my tiny, 4'10" Great Aunt Edith had already been kicked out of two assisted living facilities for wandering off and hitting a nurse. She expressed her displeasure at a third facility by dumping a dish of peaches in the hair of an unsuspecting nurse. As long as the peaches weren't in your hair, the story can be amusing in the retelling. At the time, it took all of my father's considerable powers of persuasion to convince them to keep Edith as a resident.

One cause of frustration is that most of us are used to working on

Notes

> *"Holding on to anger only gives you tense muscles."*
>
> — Joan Lunden,
> *Joan Lunden's Healthy Living*
> (New York: Crown 1997, p. 61)

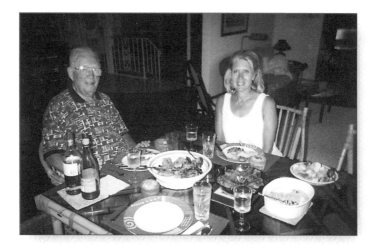

problems that improve with time and effort. Caring for children has its share of anxieties, but children eventually grow up. They get through the terrible twos, even adolescence, and become something better. Caring for an elderly person is often not a situation that gets better, except in very small increments. Aging may not be an illness, but the overall picture is often one of decline.

So, look hard for the little victories. Try not to be discouraged because her clothes don't match; focus on the fact that the person you care for is able to dress herself at all. Don't concentrate on what they forget; focus on what they can still remember even if the memories are distorted. Accepting the best you can get and the best you can do helps to lessen frustration.

"You can't stay mad at somebody who makes you laugh."

— Jay Leno

PEOPLE DON'T CHANGE

My aunt always said, "People don't change when they get older; they just become more the way they are."

To be more effective in motivating the elderly, try to remember what they were like before this point in their lives. What were their interests? Their strengths? Their weaknesses? If they were never readers, don't be surprised if they aren't interested in books when they age.

They might enjoy the social interaction of card playing instead. And, don't expect them to be nice just because they are elderly. If she wasn't a sweet young woman, she will not magically become a sweet.

N o t e s

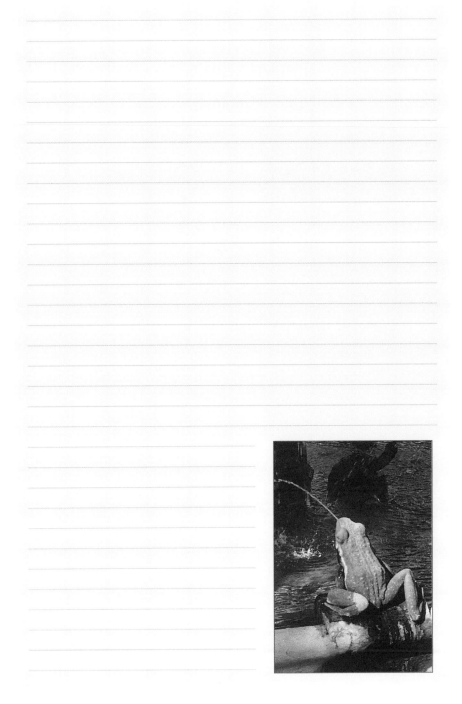

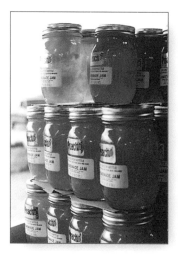

little old lady! The areas where there was friction in your relationship will probably still exist and may even be exacerbated. Can you think of some of those annoying traits as eccentricities now that they're older? They are feeling frustrated by loss of control over their own lives, and you are frustrated by the stresses of care giving!

"Never try to teach a pig to sing! It wastes your time and annoys the pig."
— Jean Marie Laskas,
"Uncommon Sense"
(The Washington Post Magazine,
April 28, 1996)

When I'm feeling frustrated that Mother is taking too long getting somewhere or doing an activity, I stop — take a breath — and smile — and hope my children will do the same for me. Next time, I should be the one to allow more time!

❤ Tips for Caregivers

❤ Find a friend who can share your "war stories" and help you laugh about them.

❤ Schedule one day a week for appointments and errands and let your elder know what day that is. It can prevent daily calls from becoming a control tactic. Non-emergency items can be kept on a running list until the next errand day.

❤ Don't ask if you don't want to hear the answer. "How are you?" is certain to lead to frustration when talking to a chronically ill person who never feels well and always tells you so. Think of another opening line! — "Good morning, what a beautiful day!"

❤ Don't be so hard on yourself.

❤ Take notes at doctors' offices. With multiple medications, doctors, appointments, symptoms and diagnoses, you can easily lose track and the patient who has seemed mentally competent in the past can be confused now.

❤ Short visits (if you can manage it) are as good as long ones.

❤ You don't need credit from others! Give yourself lots of credit by making a list of all you are doing.

Notes

DEALING WITH CONFLICTS

Some conflict is probably inevitable because elderly people often see caregivers as responsible for their losses. To reduce the frustration during these situations:

• Try to present changes as choices rather than ultimatums.

• Postpone confrontations. Many issues don't have to be dealt with immediately. Often a response of "we'll look into that" or "give me some time to think that over" will put off discussions until they can be more constructive. Sometimes problems even solve themselves!

• Provide information on a "need-to-know" basis. The full truth sometimes causes pain or anxiety and is not always necessary.

• Pick your battles. Choose issues that concern critical health and safety.

• Don't personalize.

• Accept what you cannot change.

• You only feel frustrated because you care.

"Our limited perspective, our hopes and fears become our measure of life, and when circumstances don't fit our ideas, they become our difficulties."

— Benjamin Franklin

"The process is the reality."

— Dr. Samuel Johnson

When dealing with the elderly, focus on the process, rather than concentrating on a goal.

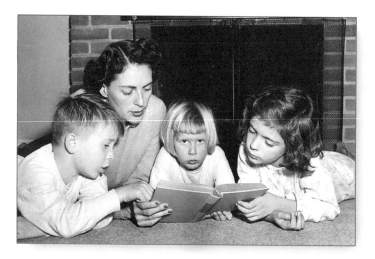

Notes

_____

_____

_____

_____

_____

_____

_____

"The world is wide, and I will not waste my life in friction when it could be turned into momentum."

— Frances Willard

 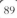

When I first mentioned to a personal friend, who worked in social services, that I would soon have both of my parents living with me in my home because of medical reasons, she immediately sat me down, looked me right in the eyes and said that the most important thing I could do for myself, my own family, and my parents would be to take care of myself. After thirteen years of care giving, I truly appreciate the value and accuracy of her advice.

CARE OF THE CAREGIVER

MEASURE YOUR JOURNEY

There is no way to know how long eldercaring responsibilities will last and how they will change in the future. Caregivers take on responsibilities that can be very time-consuming, exhausting and stressful. As you begin your care giving journey, it will help to consider ways to avoid some of the common setbacks, or roadblocks, associated with these responsibilities.

It is a fact that personal attitudes affect one's total well-being. As a caregiver you can ease stress and frustration by having a positive attitude. Since you often have little control over events and other people associated with your eldercaring, try to maintain a positive attitude, understanding, reasonable expectations and balance. To put yourself in a frame of mind that makes your task easier, it is helpful to look on your demands in a more favorable light — volunteering versus obligation, a choice to contribute rather than a responsibility, or the opportunity to return a kindness you may have received. By recognizing that you are making a conscious choice to be involved, you will be less likely to look at the task as an imposition. Consequently, you will feel more in charge.

Attitude is also influenced by understanding — the better you understand the changes associated with aging or the relevant illness, the more capable you will be in handling problems and anticipating needs. Reading and research will go a long way to prepare you. Be proactive and ask knowledgeable questions of all professionals. Questions and answers help you discover ways to make your job easier.

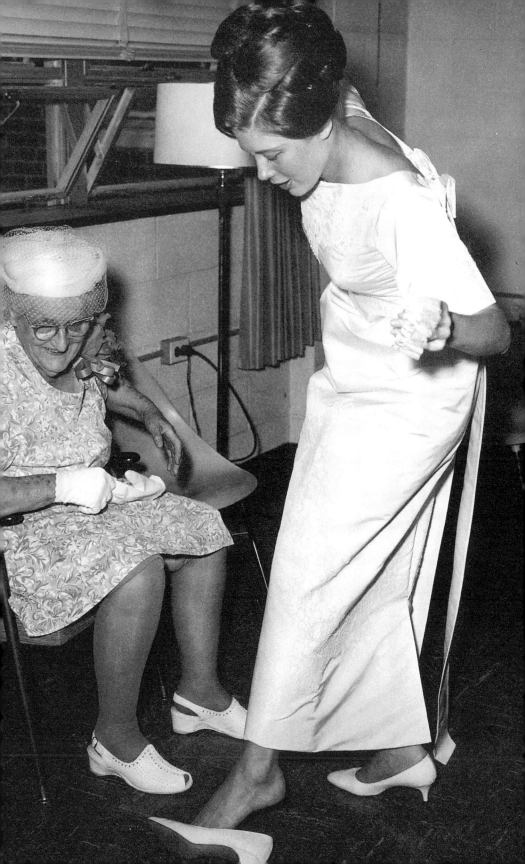

SET REASONABLE EXPECTATIONS

Setting reasonable expectations is important. If you are helping in hopes of gaining love or respect you never had, you will be disappointed. Relationships won't change now and "repaying parents" is impossible . . . parenthood is not a debt ever intended to be repaid.

Appreciation for your contributions will not necessarily be expressed.

The time and ability you have to give to eldercaring needs to be closely examined. Begin by determining if you will need to give up some of your activities. Make a list of your commitments to family members, friends, and to yourself. Then prioritize your time accordingly. Set reasonable goals. It is easier to add to your commitments at a later time, but it's harder to subtract them.

Maintaining a balance in your personal life will help you avoid

Notes

> "Our body is a well-set clock, which keeps good time, but if it be too much or indiscreetly tampered with, the alarm runs out before the hour."
>
> — Joseph Hall

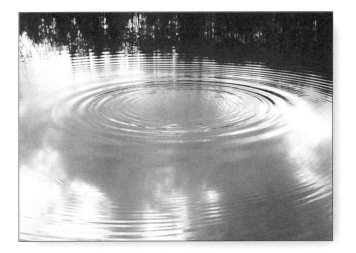

future burnout. Take time for yourself to recharge, as well as time to nurture your own family and friendships. These will become even more important to you if care giving needs increase.

Outings offer a refreshing change of scenery; activities, sports and hobbies will ease stress and provide pleasure. Pampering yourself on occasion not only reduces stress, but also helps to maintain your own self-esteem.

As a caregiver be sure to find ways to release anger and frustration: exercise, cry, express your feelings verbally or in this journal. Try not to allow yourself to take out your frustrations on your elder. If necessary, consult a counselor or find a support group that will give you the opportunity to express feelings, release stress and share information in a healthy way.

Caregivers need to look at the positive side of small nuisances, such as the need to slow down your normal pace when accompanying your elder (we often miss out on the fine points of life by being in too much of a rush, anyway). Make a point of seeing the glass as "half full" as opposed to "half empty." A bad mood or attitude will only make your job harder. A sense of humor and positive approach contribute to good personal health. Above all, congratulate yourself on handling new challenges. Self-satisfaction is its own reward.

PLEASANTRIES

My mother, whose Alzheimer's was in the early stage, was living at home with a wonderful companion. Her doctor recommended that she go to the Senior

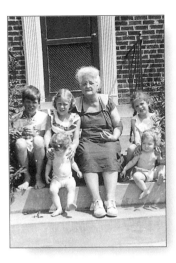

Citizens Day Care, run by the local government, to have more interaction with other people. I drove her there her first day and she said, "If you leave me here, I'll kill myself." I answered, "Well, if that's what you want, do it here rather than at home — it'd be easier." With dementia, sometimes agreeing or distracting makes more sense than arguing. When Mother got inside, her social side prevailed and she loved her stay.

❤ Tips to Keep Healthy

❤ Protect your own health. . . you'll need it more than ever. Stay active. Physical activity prevents disease and is a great reliever of stress and depression.

❤ Don't wear yourself out with unnecessary tasks. Select carefully where you will expend your energy.

❤ Simplify — simplify — simplify.

❤ Get enough sleep. When you are rested, you are a far better caregiver and are more pleasant to be around!

❤ Breaks energize. Take time off to recharge.

❤ Take time to sit down and eat nutritious meals.

❤ Tips for Peace of Mind

❤ Try not to be disappointed when expectations are not met and gratitude is not expressed. Learn to pat yourself on the back and take pride in your own accomplishments.

❤ Keeping a journal of your thoughts, good and bad, can be cathartic.

❤ A brisk walk relieves anger.

❤ Music, whether soothing or lively, can make tasks more enjoyable.

❤ Join a support group for advice and information as well as for emotional support.

❤ Talking to friends, your pastor or a counselor can help ease the burdens. We acquire courage and comfort from good friends who stand by us and support us.

❤ Don't neglect your personal life. Keep in touch with friends and continue personal interests and activities. Conserve time by combining exercise or activities with time spent with friends or family.

♥ Creating and maintaining a positive attitude will go a long way toward keeping healthy. People who are depressed are more likely to have health problems than people with happy outlooks on life. Cheerfulness helps to keep one's energy level high.

♥ Doctors recognize that laughter is beneficial to one's health. It is an often forgotten healer. It is okay to laugh, no matter how sick or incompetent your elder may be. In fact, the worse things get, the more you should seek things to laugh about.

Notes

> "The most wasted of all days is that during which one has not laughed."
>
> — Nicolas Chamfort, *Timeless Wisdom* (Cake Eaters, Inc., 1994, p. 23)
>
> "In the end, everything is a gag."
>
> — Charlie Chaplin

♥ TIPS TO RELIEVE STRESS

♥ Practice relaxation techniques when you feel yourself becoming tense. There are many books available that will help you.

♥ Do not hesitate to say "no" if the task is not absolutely necessary. Being a healthy "hero" is better than being a burned-out "super hero".

♥ When frustrated by your elder, leave the room for a few minutes to regain your composure.

♥ Sticking to a schedule will help you feel more in control. A forgotten item at the store can usually wait for the next trip.

♥ Let your employer know about your eldercaring responsibilities and inquire about the possibility of a more flexible work schedule.

♥ Acknowledge your emotions and find an outlet for them. You will undoubtedly experience anxiety, worry for your elder, guilt, sadness, resentment and anger. These emotions are normal so don't hesitate to discuss them with friends.

♥ Rather than being upset when expectations are not met, lower expectations. Be realistic in the goals you set for yourself and your elder.

♥ The more unrewarding the activity, the higher the chance for burnout. The more intimate the care, the more stressful it is.

♥ Let the telephone answering machine give you a break.

"My candle burns at both ends; It will not last the night."

— Edna St. Vincent Millay

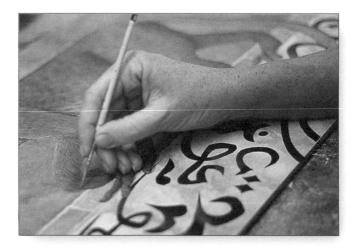

Notes

> "God give us the grace to accept with serenity the things that cannot be changed, courage to change the things that should be changed, and the wisdom to distinguish the one from the other."
>
> — Reinhold Niebuhr, "The Serenity Prayer"

♥ TIPS TO NOURISH HEART AND SOUL

♥ If you and your parents live together, you can still have a social life; just be a little more flexible. Leave your parent at home with a sitter or invite friends in for a potluck supper where each guest brings a course and you're not cooking everything.

♥ If your elder is in a care facility, preparing ahead will make your visits more rewarding. *The Brown University Long-Term Care Quality Letter* (May 16, 1994 , vol. 6) suggests planning an activity such as a manicure or taking a "prop" such as a photo album to prompt reminiscence. Planning your departure prior to a meal or other absorbing activity is suggested to ease the separation.

♥ Recognize that you do not have to do it all. Being a good caregiver does not require that you become a martyr. Accepting help from others will help prevent burnout.

♥ Adult daycare and visiting nurses will offer a daytime break. Respite care is available in some localities for overnight assistance. Check your elder into a nursing home or private facility for a vacation from eldercaring.

♥ Extend care to other caregivers (such as a hired, live-in aide) by relieving them for an hour, an afternoon or an overnight. This will acknowledge that they need a break and will show that their welfare is being considered as well as their patient's.

Notes

> *"A merry heart doeth good like a medicine; but a broken spirit drieth the bones"*
>
> — Proverbs 17:22

I'm in an airplane right now en route to my home in Arlington, Texas having just left Denver where I've spent the last three days with Mother and Dad. My heart is heavy as I realize that Mother, who is experiencing ever increasing difficulties with dementia, just can't cope any more, and frankly right now I can't cope with my mother.

RESOURCES FOR LONG DISTANCE CARE

An ever-increasing number of Americans are dealing with "long distance" care giving of older relatives. By its very nature, long distance elder-caring is complex and challenging. What resources are available? How can transportation be obtained? Do they have food? Are the bills being paid? What will happen if an emergency should arise? These are just a few of the many questions and situations that arise for long distance caregivers. An important first step is to call Eldercare Locator, a service of the federal government, which will guide you to the local senior services available in any part of the country (800-677-1116). Other agencies are available, such as the National Association of Area Agencies on Aging (202-296-8130), or Children of Aging Parents (800-227-7294).

There are an increasing number of excellent home healthcare services available. Naturally, extreme care should be given to selecting the right service or providers since abuse and fraud are known to exist, but such services can help the elderly remain in their own homes as long as possible. Home healthcare providers supply nursing services; occupational and physical therapists provide dressing and bathing aids and help with housekeeping chores. A new profession called Geriatric-Care Managers (GCM) is another source for long distance caregivers. A GCM is an on-site family proxy who can arrange and oversee care, services and companionship. A GCM may charge anywhere from $50 to $150 per hour.

Many more services are inexpensive or free. Grocery stores offer delivery services for a nominal fee. Groceries, flowers, medical supplies, and household sundries can be

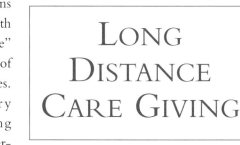

LONG DISTANCE CARE GIVING

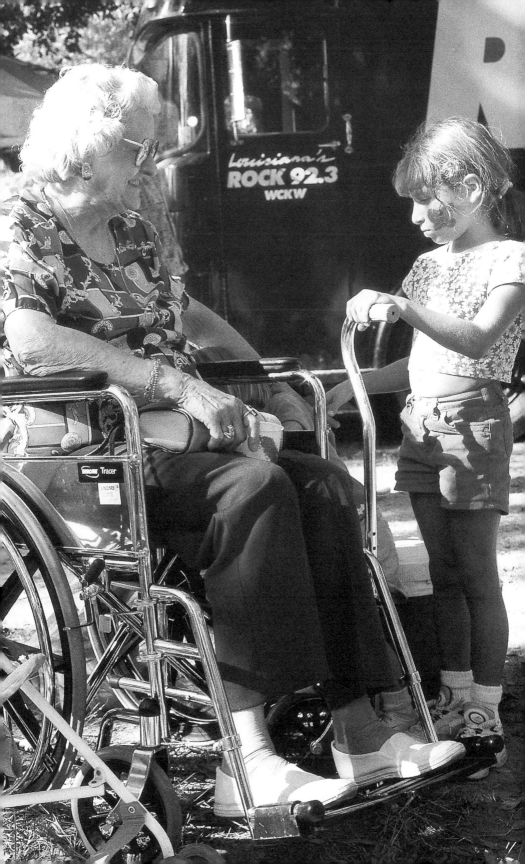

ordered by the caregiver from afar and delivered to an older person who is unable to manage or plan a week's worth of menus and who may also have difficulty with transportation. The caregiver is also able to play an important role by promoting good nutrition. Make sure a wide variety of healthy foods are available. There are also hot meal services that the long distance caregiver can call on for help.

Organizations like Meals on Wheels, a private, nonprofit corporation provides hot lunches to the elderly or disabled. Susan Chappel, the director of the Arlington, Texas program says: "The benefit of the program isn't just nutritional. Daily human contact improves the emotional well being of the clients who live alone. The main thing is someone checks on them everyday."

It is important for the long distance caregiver to establish good relationships with people who have frequent contact with their elder. The next door neighbor, the senior's friends, the visiting nurse or housekeeper, the minister — all can act

Notes

as your "eyes and ears" and keep you informed of any changes in behavior or health. Make sure they have your home and work phone numbers, and that they feel comfortable calling you. Visit with them each time you're in town, and let them know how much you appreciate their generous help.

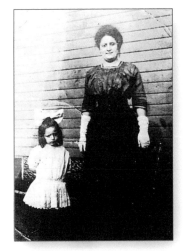

Even with your best intentions and help from a variety of sources, plan on making visits as frequently as possible. The elderly are easy prey for unscrupulous telemarketers or door-to-door scams, sweepstakes come-ons, theft and abuse. Discuss the possibility of frauds and scams with your loved ones. Keep in mind, however, that dementia, depression, and loneliness can lead to poor decisions or the inability to deal with complex business or financial situations.

MAKING THE DECISION

I call Mom and Dad to check on them frequently. One day I asked if they had had their lunch. Mom hesitated, obviously confused. Then, after a brief moment, she replied, "Oh yes — we had soup. I just found the empty soup can in the trash." Even when you call, you can't be sure things are going correctly!

The rise in long distance eldercaring is a predictable consequence of our mobile society. The increasing number of elderly adults requiring care and the greater distance separating them from their adult children (those usually most willing to help), offers a challenge that can be extremely frustrating and at times frightening.

The key to long distance care is mapping out plans early. Experts warn against putting off painful discussions and decisions. The worst time to do the planning is when there is a crisis. Do not let "long distance" be the excuse.

Reaching a consensus may be the most difficult part because of differences in each individual's perception of the circumstances. Children are often more concerned with such issues as physical limitations, financial accountability and emotional needs, while their parents' primary focus may be on maintaining some degree of autonomy, dignity and independence.

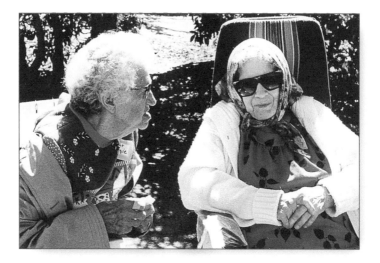

Assessing the needs and the support systems already in place should be the first step before uprooting a parent. Identify informal support networks, such as neighbors and friends, community service organizations and churches.

SELECTING A LOCATION — YOUR PLACE OR MINE?

Are you considering moving your parents to live nearby? Be aware that elderly people may become seriously depressed after moving to a new location, even if the purpose is to be closer to their children. *When my mother-in-law moved from Arizona to Virginia, we found that not only was she depressed, but her dogs were too!*

Changes like eating in a large dining facility and making new friends can be a huge adjustment. Suspect depression if they spend an inordinate amount of time sleeping or sitting in front of a television.

Before making the transition, be sure that your expectations for your parents meet their needs, wants and abilities. A parent who has always preferred more individual activities such as reading, gardening and needlework, is not going to suddenly change into a golf or tennis enthusiast. Likewise, a parent who has always loved outdoor activities will be extremely unhappy cooped up in a small apartment in a location with long and treacherous winters.

N o t e s

> "You gain strength,
> courage and confidence
> by every experience in
> which you really stop to
> look fear in the face."
>
> — Eleanor Roosevelt

Whenever you are moving your parent to an assisted care setting for senior citizens or placing them in a more institutional setting, such as a nursing home, you must investigate the facility's track record. Many times care facilities for the elderly have different priorities and agendas. Eldercare facilities are expensive. It is usually in the best interest of the facility to keep your loved one on as a resident. Therefore, it is very important that you or someone nearby continue to monitor whether or not the facility is able to provide the services required.

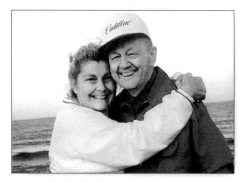

Before you decide on placement in a nursing care setting, there are several guidelines to follow:

• Ask for references,

• Obtain a copy of the state licensing survey,

• Visit the location several times and at different times (i.e. evenings, weekends, holidays),

• Ask if the facility provides individual care plans,

• Request information about the staff-to-patient ratio,

• Then check it out yourself, and continue to be vigilant.

Consider getting an 800 phone number

Let your parents know they can call you at any time (your kids, too!). The 800 number comes in handy when you are asking health professionals, community service people, neighbors, etc. to call you back to talk regarding your parent's situation or condition. Set up specific times and days of the week for telephone communication.

Send photos frequently

When far from your loved ones who cannot visit frequently, send pictures of family, home, your activities and your children (even the dog). Always get double prints made of your pictures. Do not send the entire set at once, but send two or three with every correspondence. Send the best pictures already framed or in a photo magnet for the refrigerator. Seniors have trouble getting out to purchase frames, so the pictures may be set aside and lost. Write on the back of photos who, what, where and when, so the elder person can refresh his memory.

N o t e s

Make a video of special occasions

If you have a video camera and your loved ones know how to work a VCR or have a helper who can, a video can be a powerful tool. Not only can it make special occasions come to life for the senior citizen who could not be there, but it can be used in other ways. Your elder can use the tape to "participate" in a family activity such as exercising together, singing together of old favorites, or praying together.

Go shopping together from long distance

Order household items and clothing from catalogs. Send a duplicate set of catalogs to your parent(s). Then look through them together by phone to make selections. Have the elder's credit card number so you can do the ordering. This works well when choosing gifts for grandchildren, too. Catalogs like Speigel, J.C. Penney, Orvis and Land's End are good to have. Sears has a catalog with health care needs.

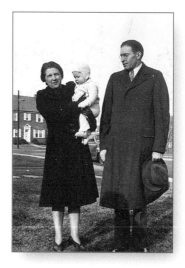

MAINTAINING YOUR OWN SANITY

There will be times when you simply cannot do it alone. Remember to share the eldercaring. AARP's Health Advocacy Services has put together an 18-page booklet, *Miles Away and Still Caring*, devoted specifically to the concerns of long-distance caregivers. The booklet includes a care-management worksheet, suggested assistance, reading materials, and community resources. For the free Caregiver Resource Kit (DI5267), address a postcard to the title and number, AARP Fulfillment (EE0756), P.O. Box 22796, Long Beach, CA 90801-5796. Allow four to six weeks for delivery.

"The heart never becomes wrinkled."

— Mme. De Sevigne

Despite all the support systems that have been put in place, there are going to be times when your frustrations, anxiety levels and comfort zones demand that you go see your loved one for yourself. To get the most accurate appraisal of the situation, plan an unannounced visit. Make the most of your time during the visit to make contact with the bank, physicians, neighbors and other caregivers.

Time is one of life's most important commodities. Caring for our parents, even from a long distance, can occupy our time whether it be physical or simply emotional. If we allow ourselves to be consumed with care giving of our elderly loved ones, we may be sacrificing a part of ourselves and taking time away from our own immediate family members. If we are not careful, our "caring" can adversely affect our relationships with co-workers, children and spouses.

If your priorities get a little out of whack, get some help for yourself. There are support groups in your community with other caregivers which provide an outlet from your frustrations, offer alternative solutions to problems, and, more importantly, provide comfort and understanding. You'll find these groups in your telephone directory or under the health or community calendar sections of the newspaper.

❤ **TIPS FOR THE CAREGIVER**
- ❤ Create boundaries.
- ❤ Stop trying to please everyone.
- ❤ Never make a promise you can't keep.
- ❤ Keep it simple.
- ❤ Strive for realistic deadlines.
- ❤ Set achievable goals.
- ❤ Approach problems as challenges.

When You Are Old

How many loved your moments of glad grace,
And loved your beauty, with love false or true,
But one man loved the pilgrim soul in you,
And loved the sorrows of your changing face.

— William Butler Yeats (1893)

"That best portion of
a good man's life,
His little nameless,
unremembered acts
Of kindness and of love."

— William Wordsworth

*M*other has always enjoyed entertaining and would take special care with her appearance. Age and macular degeneration have caused dramatic changes for her. One afternoon Mother was ready to have dinner with friends, and I noticed her dress was stained in the front. Not being able to see this because of her poor vision, Mother eagerly greeted her guests. Rather than bring the unsightly stains to her attention in front of company, I privately suggested that she put on a sweater to go with her outfit; we would worry about the stains later. I know Mother appreciated my efforts to protect her dignity.

WITH DIGNITY COMES SELF-WORTH

Feelings of dignity breed self-esteem. In the rush and fuss of your fast-paced lifestyle, don't forget your aging loved one's feelings of self-worth. Maintaining and protecting his or her dignity is an important role in eldercaring. This may be done out of pure love, or simply because we know that it is the right thing to do. Every person needs to be respected and treated as a worthy human being. As caregivers, we may need to realize that we are participants in maintaining the dignity of our elderly.

DIGNITY

How can the caregiver help to promote the elder person's self-esteem? To a great extent, this will depend on his or her physical and mental condition. In advanced cases of dementia and Alzheimer's Disease, the elder's awareness of events may be so lacking that the caregiver is the sole keeper and protector of dignity. Adult respect is challenging when dementia strikes. Even while cutting food or bathing, remember, this person is not a child and does not deserve to be treated like one. This person has lived a long life, had dreams, felt broken-hearted, felt pleasures and a wealth of experiences — even if not remembered — and deserves adult respect. Remember it is the disease causing the behaviors and lack of consciousness. Protect dignity, champion modesty, and demand that others do the same.

On the other hand, for the elder who is still alert, aware, and able to function reasonably well physically, respect can be shown with common courtesies. Never regard persons as invisible by talking over the top of their heads or by referring to them in the third person when they are present. The elderly person who is ignored will feel invisible. It is

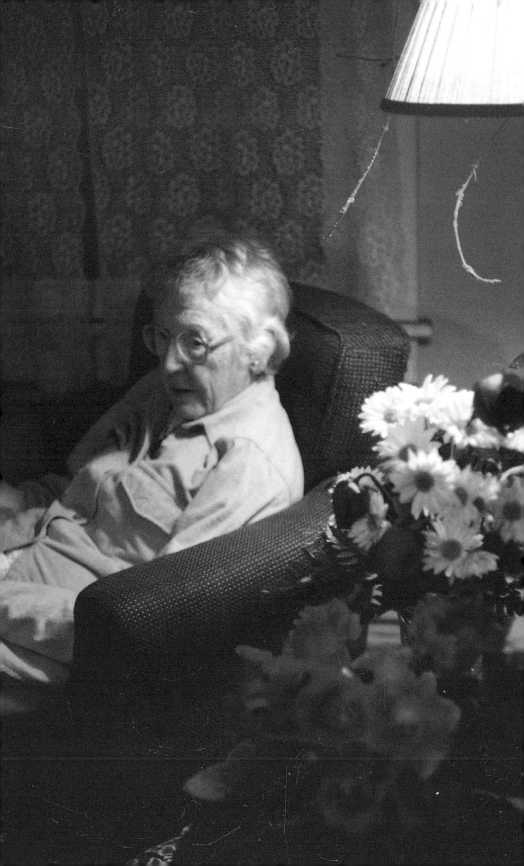

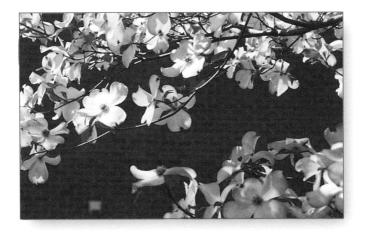

important to address the elderly directly, and encourage others to do likewise, including everyone in group conversations. Never compare the elder to a child. Be the guardian of respect. If others act or speak disrespectfully, put their behaviors in perspective and set about rebuilding their essential feelings of self-worth and dignity.

LOOKING AND FEELING GOOD

Find a level at which the elderly person will feel self-worth and encourage it. Does she still have a good sense of humor, a good memory of sports, an interest in books or current events, or stories about long-ago youth? Revisit her younger years with family albums; help her record childhood or family stories in a memory book or on tape. Pay compliments and show appreciation for expertise wherever it may be.

There is a certain sense of well-being in a clean and attractive appearance, for all human beings. Helping the elderly person to maintain cleanliness and an attractive appearance will do a great deal to promote feelings of self-esteem. Remember — happy minutes each hour and small positive feelings each day can add up to living life with dignity and well-being.

Most importantly, treat them as we ourselves would want to be treated in their circumstances. The motivation to safeguard their dignity may be in knowing that it is the right thing to do.

Notes

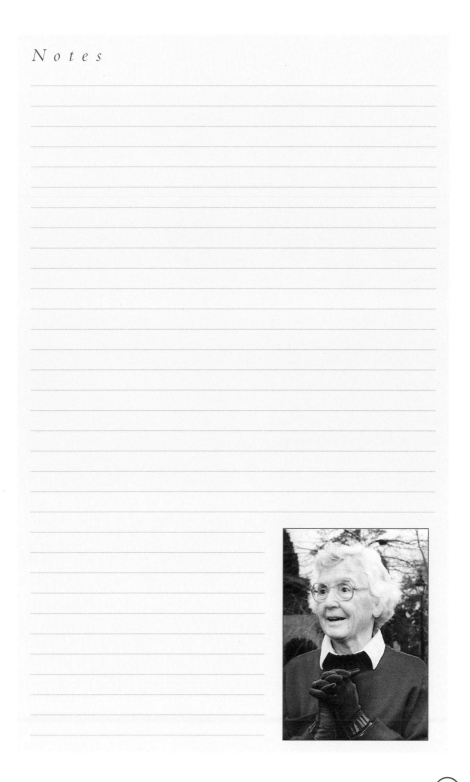

♥ TIPS FOR TREATING THE ELDERLY WITH DIGNITY

My father taught me many wonderful things in my life; the last being that death is part of the whole amazing process of being born, of loving, of living and of dying.

♥ Give the elderly an opportunity to help with household chores such as setting the table or folding laundry. The task may not be done perfectly, but they will feel involved and useful.

♥ When a waiter asks you what your elderly guest wants to eat, respond by saying, "Mother, what would you like?" Being old doesn't make one deaf.

♥ Plan ahead to avoid disasters that are embarrassing. If spilling is a problem, serve soup in a mug rather than a bowl. Serve meats that are easy to cut or pre-cut in the kitchen. Keep clutter out of pathways to prevent falls.

♥ Respond to elders when they speak, even if it's just a nod. You wouldn't ignore the words of a friend. Make sure your tone of voice is not condescending.

♥ If elders ask your opinion about their appearance, respond with an attitude that indcates you care about their pride in themselves.

♥ Hospitals tend to strip people of their dignity. Insist that the hospital staff tell the elder what is being done to them and why. Ask the staff to address your elder by the title or name to which he or she is accustomed, Mr., Mrs., Major. Protect modesty with an appropriate nightgown or robe. Be sure curtains are drawn when necessary. Deal firmly with difficult roommates.

> *"When we seek to discover the best in others, we somehow bring out the best in ourselves."*
>
> — William Arthur Ward

N o t e s

KEEPING UP

Joan's mother is always saying, "I don't feel like I belong in the world anymore." Perhaps that feeling of isolation is inevitable, when elders no longer understand the humor of the day or the manners and morals around them. However, helping them keep abreast of current events may increase their comfort in a society that continues to speed by while they are slowing down.

Access to a television or radio seems like it would be sufficient, but many elderly people never turn them on. In that case, reading the paper to them for fifteen minutes will make them feel that they are still involved in the world. Most people enjoy being read to and the benefit is, of course, twofold. The elderly person is exposed to the news and also enjoys attention from the caregiver. If the material is well chosen, both will enjoy the process.

Warmth and love are powerful. When the elderly become anxious, depressed, or riled, stroke their hand or cheek. A gentle touch will help both of you get through the moment.

Notes

Never Underestimate Your Parents' Abilities

Friends of mine, a couple, went to considerable and inconvenient lengths to hide from her failing mother that they were living together though they were not married. At least once a year her mother would come to town and the man would essentially move out, hiding all evidence of his residence in the apartment. After more than three years of this nuisance, before the next visit of the elderly mother, the couple finally telephoned to announce that they were engaged to marry. At this the mother said, "But wait, have you considered living together for awhile first?"

Maybe, too frequently, we underestimate the abilities of the older generation to "keep up with the times." Failing physically does not necessarily mean failing awareness or inflexibility.

"There is dignity in allowing people to make choices, and take risks."
— Clara Pratt, Director of Oregon State University's Gerontology Program, quoted by Betty Friedan, *The Fountain of Age.* (New York: Simon & Schuster. 1993, p. 528-529)

> *"Take care of your parents — Your children may be watching!"*
> — Anonymous
> Bumper Sticker

Solutions for Maintaining Independence

The elderly often feel that they are no longer looked upon with respect because they have to ask others to perform many of the tasks of daily living. Fortunately, there is a wide selection of helpful devices available that can prolong independence, dignity, and self-worth.

There have been many improvements in the products that promote mobility:

• Canes can be collapsible and carried unobtrusively when not in use. They also come with four prongs for stability.

• There are motorized scooters and wheelchairs with all kinds of accessories.

• For the elder who needs support but doesn't require a wheelchair, there is a wonderful innovation that resembles a walk-behind stool on four wheels. It has a seat if the user needs to stop for a rest and a basket for carrying packages (or laundry). Since they don't have to be lifted up like a walker, the user can move faster and with less effort, saving precious energy for other activities. They are also equipped with hand brakes and come in jazzy, metallic colors. *My mother-in-law calls it her Cadillac. It has become the status symbol that the real thing was in her driving days.*

• Steps are often a major hindrance to independence. To address this problem there are half-height stairs to adapt regular eight-inch risers to a manageable height.

• Stair lifts and even home elevators can be installed to maintain independence.

• Kitchen accessories and special tableware for those with hand tremors can make it possible for the elderly to feed themselves. Counters and cabinets can be raised and lowered by elevators at the touch of a button. "Reachers" for extending arthritic or weakened arms can be purchased in different lengths and with batteries to open and close the jaws for gripping.

• Adjustable electric beds, lift chairs and swivel seats not only provide comfort but may allow the elderly to move around without asking for assistance. Bathroom safety products like raised commodes, shower seats and safety rails can mean a protection of basic privacy and maintain dignity. Talking watches and bedside clocks are available through mail-order and local stores. Just press a button, and the time is read aloud.

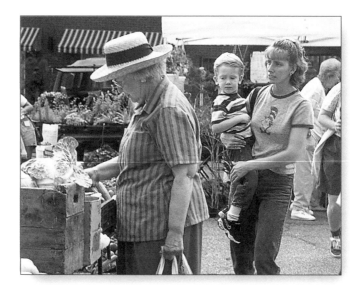

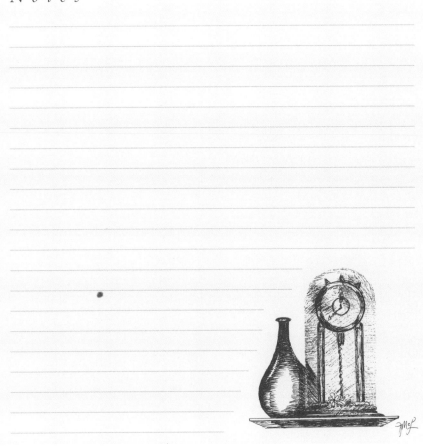

• Aids for putting on socks, elastic shoelaces that don't need to be tied and extended shoehorns are helpful for those who cannot easily reach their feet when dressing.

• Elastic waists and Velcro closings are much easier than buttons.

Together with the advice of health professionals (particularly physical and occupational therapists) the improvements in equipment for the elderly can greatly increase independence. More independence will improve their quality of life and sense of dignity. Check to see whether the cost of these aids is covered by Medicare or supplemental insurance. They may be tax deductible if not covered.

GIVE CREDIT
WHERE CREDIT IS DUE!

At a funeral I attended recently, I was touched by the son who gave the eulogy for his mother. In it he said, "The family is especially grateful for my mother's guardian angel, the caregiver at the nursing home where she lived for fifteen years. By her thoughtfulness and devotion, she was able to give Mother dignity up until the end."

MANAGING INCONTINENCE

Incontinence is a cruel thief of dignity. It can have many causes, but may prove to be a chronic problem; and, like many of the infirmities of old age, you may just have to manage it in the best ways you can. Talking with your elder is the only way to ease the humiliation that accompanies incontinence. Find solutions through this gentle, sympathetic and tactful conversation.

♥ **KEEP THESE TIPS IN MIND:**

♥ Arrange for a medical evaluation. Determine what is causing the incontinence and whether or not it can be helped by medication or surgery.

♥ Try to insure that the bathroom is always accessible. If the bathroom is not shared, it will be free when needed. Provide a portable commode or bedpan if necessary.

> *"High station in life is earned by the gallantry with which appalling experiences are survived with grace."*
>
> — Tennessee Williams,
> *Memoirs* (New York: Doubleday)

Avoid going to places where accessibility is difficult or nonexistent. Choose seats in restaurants and other public places that are near restrooms (call ahead to make arrangements and avoid embarrassment).

♥ Equip the bathroom with appropriate aids. A raised commode and grab bars can make trips to the bathroom easier when speed is critical.

♥ Encourage wearing clothes that are easy to manage: knee-highs rather than pantyhose, Velcro fasteners rather than buttons, washable clothes rather than those that need dry cleaning.

♥ Restrict liquids after 5 p.m.

♥ Be sure that the bladder is emptied before going to bed.

♥ Experiment with timed voiding. Attempting to empty the bladder every two to three hours during the night (when more urine is produced) reduces the risk of losing control. This may require setting an alarm.

♥ Use waterproof pads on beds and chairs. Pads can be purchased in disposable or washable form and can be improvised by placing a shower curtain liner inside a folded sheet.

♥ Diaper-like products for adults are readily available. Experi-ment to find the type that seems to work best.

♥ Reduce odors by providing a small, lidded pail with a deodorizer for storing soiled clothes and bedding until they can be laundered. Maintain a supply of room deodorizing sprays; an open box of baking soda can also help rid a room of odors.

N o t e s

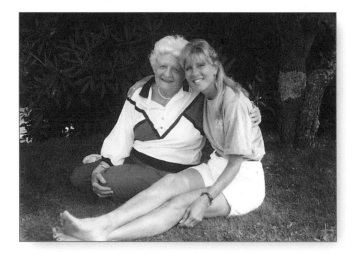

GROOMING

Encouraging good grooming is important for the health and self-esteem of the elderly. Regular appointments and shopping for new clothes provide outings and special occasions they can anticipate. The elderly still enjoy a good time!

If appearance used to be very important to your loved one, consider doing a little extra out of respect for the grooming standards they once held.

One friend, to whom appearance is very important, has gone a step further and maintains her mother-in-law up to her own standards. Even though clothes were never that important to her mother-in-law, in her 80's she loves the extra attention and understands that it is a visible sign of her daughter-in-law's love for her.

Periodically, however, you may need to reassess the level of personal grooming that is appropriate. Routines that were once desirable may no longer be possible or sensible.

Organize closets to make it easier for the elderly:

• Hang all the pieces to an outfit on the same hanger and label it. Include the appropriate shoes on the shelf right above.

• Rotate the order of clothes on the closet rod. This may encourage them to reach for different outfits.

• Provide sweaters and lightweight jackets that are in neutral colors and will complement many outfits. The elderly are often cold and require layers to remain comfortable.

• Arrange regular appointments for hair and nail care. Pedicures may be important for health and

N o t e s

By the time my father-in-law entered the nursing home, it was clear that disease had taken its toll on both his body and mind. We quickly realized that our visits would often begin with the unexpected. Sometimes he would be walking in the hall or perhaps trying to take a nap in someone else's bed and become quite irate that the fellow who was already in the bed refused to move. On one occasion we arrived when he was threatening bodily harm with his cane to the nurse who simply wanted him to return to his own room. Always polite and reserved, this was un-characteristic behavior. Even though I realized he was acting strangely, I was not pre-pared to find him on our next visit sit-ting at the table in his room naked from the waist down. My mother-in-law was embarrassed, but he seemed unaware that anything was amiss. So I took my cue from him and just said, "My, it looks like you've forgotten something. Let's get some pants on, it's cold in here."

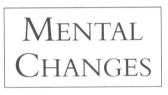

MENTAL CHANGES

PHYSICAL CHANGES

Alzheimer's Disease and related forms of dementia affect behavior as well as intellect. In fact, some of the earliest signs of the disease can be subtle changes in personality and social behavior. Our "social antennae," of course, rely on intact cerebral function. Degenerative or post-traumatic damage to the brain can result in a loss of inhibition, so that the patient exhibits anti-social behavior such as inappropriate lan-guage, often with a sexual content. Patients can react with aggressive outbursts over even minor frustra-tions. Grooming may deteriorate. Some patients may even appear nude in public surroundings with-out embarrassment. All of these changes are related to the loss of brain cells and accompanying neuro-chemical changes in the brain. It is these personality changes that are the most stressful for caregivers since the patient now appears to be "a different person." Support groups for care-givers offer an opportunity to share these experiences with others.

Confide in your doctor when these changes occur. It is important to provide a list of all strange behav-iors before an office visit so the doctor is able to review the infor-mation ahead of time. It is often difficult or impossible to talk about changes in behaviors in front of the patient during consultation. One strategy for a caregiver is to have the secretary put a Post-it™ note on the front of the chart requesting a con-fidential moment with the doctor.

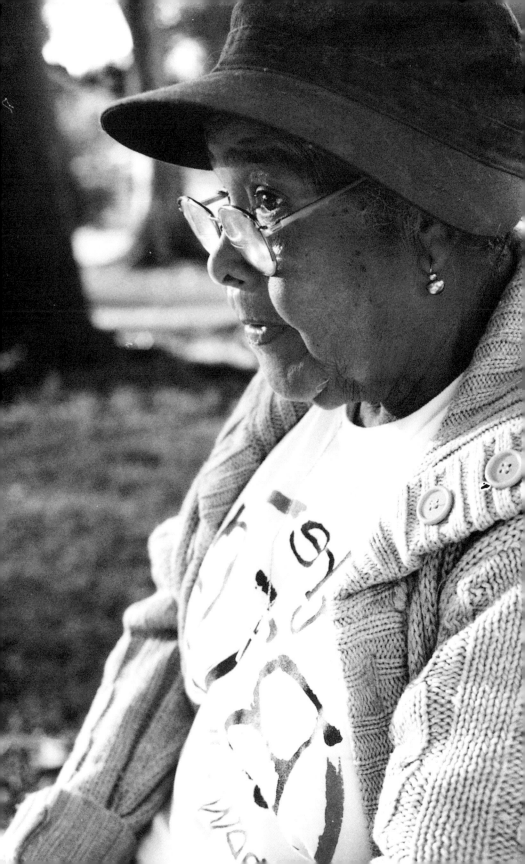

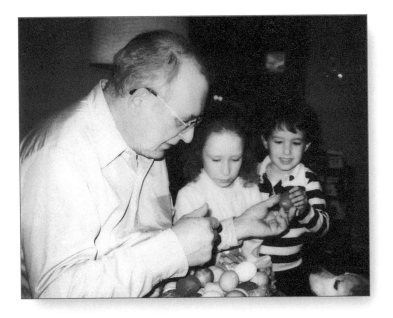

NEVER SAY NEVER!

"Mother, I promise never to put you in a nursing home."

Those words may well come back to haunt you. Instead say, "I promise to take care of you as well as I can." Situations change and you cannot always do what you would like.

Because of the aggressive, even violent, behavior that sometimes comes with Alzheimer's Disease, my mother's physician directed that she be placed in an Alzheimer's unit. It was no longer safe for her to be cared for at home.

You may never find the perfect place for your loved one but if you are flexible and open you may encourage him or her to be the same. One woman living in a suite with another widow while waiting for a private room to become available found that she enjoyed the companionship of her new friend. She elected to remain in the suite instead of moving when she had the opportunity. Another lady confided to visitors that she had decided not to live with her daughter because she recognized the strain it would place on the family. She was able to think of it as her own wise decision, without resentment and feelings of rejection. It doesn't matter who realized that the retirement home would be a better place for her to live. Daily calls and enthusiastic visits reassured her of her family's love.

Notes

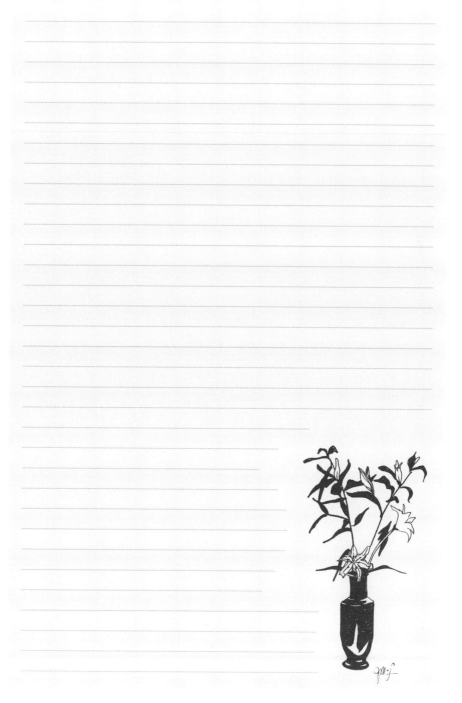

Notes

_____

_____

_____

_____

_____

_____

_____

_____

_____

_____

_____

_____

_____

THE BALM OF COMPANIONSHIP

My 87-year-old grandmother had a stroke which left her partially paralyzed and unable to speak. She was placed in a nursing home in the small town where she had lived all of her life, and my mother was able to visit her every day. Grandmother rarely expressed any emotion except when she saw a friend. As Mother wheeled her through the halls, she would see an old friend, reach out and squeeze her hand and give her the best smile she could. Even without the exchange of words, those instances seemed to bring her such joy. The sad part, however, is that her best friend could not bring herself to visit Grandmother in the nursing home (she couldn't bear to see Grandmother in that state). I know that even a five-minute visit every once in awhile would have meant so much to Grandmother during her seven-year stay.

Well-intentioned friends and relatives often find it difficult to visit stroke or Alzheimer's patients who may speak unintelligibly, show few signs of understanding their surroundings, or don't even recognize their loved ones. The presence of other patients with whom they do not have caring relationships can make it even more difficult, depressing or even frightening.

THE TEACHABLE MOMENT

When my mother was in the Alzheimer's unit of an assisted living home, our family got together every week at my brother's home which was not far away. Mother was included in the evening, too, and it was a happier setting for everyone. Although Mother was only able to communicate with noises, we pretended we knew what she was trying to say. Once my five-year-old niece had a friend over who appeared to be frightened by Mother. But my niece turned to her and said, "Don't worry; that's just how Grandma talks."

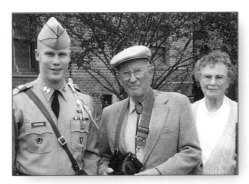

Sometimes props like photographs make visits easier. If they stimulate some reaction from the patient, it is easier to respond, even if it is just a guess as to what they are actually saying. Try dressing up for visits. Women patients, particularly, seem to react to what their visitors are wearing. Perhaps they instinctively feel it is a special occasion.

THE RIGHT PLACE TO MOVE?

Grandfather was not a happy camper when it became necessary to move him to a nursing home. He would yell out constantly that he didn't want to be there. The staff moved him several times, finally settling on a room shared by a very polite gentleman named Reginald who left the room to give us privacy during our visit. When we left, Mother said to him, "You can go back to your room now." Reginald replied, "What did you say?" Mother responded, "Do you want to go to bed?" "Oh, yes," replied Reginald, "How much do you charge?" As you can imagine, the nursing staff doubled over with laughter and we realized why this was the perfect room for Grandfather . . . it was shared with a deaf roommate!

Don't give up on finding solutions for living arrangements. The decision you make may not be what you were positive was the answer when you began the process. A doctor confided that he had been determined to move his elderly mother from Minnesota to the warmth of Arizona. But after a miserable year in Phoenix, he realized that she was better off in familiar surroundings and moved her back to a retirement home in her old neighborhood. He had the difficulties of long-distance elder-caring but felt it was the right decision for them.

My grandmother made a difficult move from her home in the Southwest to an assisted living facility in Virginia where our family could take better care of her. She was not always happy to be here, but at her death a year later I realized it was a good move. My sister and I came to know and love her in a way that we never could have had she remained two thousand miles away. I think she knew it, too. I hope so.

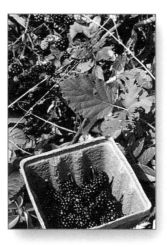

EXPECT THE UNEXPECTED!

Mother hid items in her underwear drawer and she kept food under her bed.

When visiting the Alzheimer's unit one day, I saw a resident wearing Mother's pretty flowered dress. Knowing that "borrowing each other's clothes" is symptomatic, I complimented her on her good taste rather than making a fuss. Her dress would end up back in her own closet by the end of the day.

Some dementia patients get pleasure from routine chores, such as mowing the lawn — even if the chores aren't essential. It can be therapeutic for them. One patient mowed the lawn daily. Another patient continually put on more and more clothes ending up with multiple layers. It was necessary for his spouse to put out daily outfits for him. Another woman continued to do well with her card games despite her difficulties in other areas.

Aunt Alyda had always been a fashionable dresser with a passion for expensive gold jewelry. When she had to be moved to a nursing home, the family presented her with a pretty costume jewelry "gold" bracelet to substitute for her real one. At once, she reverted to her flamboyant style of using her hands while speaking! She derived much pleasure in wearing that bracelet and it was with her to the end. Perhaps she didn't even realize it wasn't her usual 14k quality.

> *"The greatest good you can do for another is not just to share your riches, but to reveal to him his own."*
>
> — Benjamin Disraeli

Notes

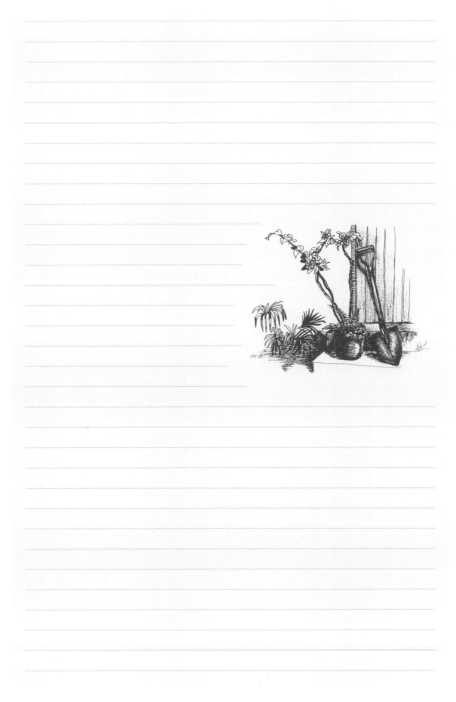

Having just sent a class of fifth graders home for the summer, I drove over to my parents' retirement community to pick up my dad . . . as planned, he was going to live with me for the summer. Dad was fast approaching the later stages of Parkinson's disease; he was frail, very unsteady, experiencing incontinence, and confusion. Mom's own condition of macular degeneration prevented her from caring for Dad at this stage. A week later, after moving Mom into a small apartment, helping her adjust to being alone for the first time in 52 years, and settling Dad into a routine that required my twenty-four-hour attention, I knew I needed help in a BIG way. I discovered the Visiting Nurses Association. This organization was a godsend for all three of us. The VNA offered home care for Dad, counseling for Mom, support and time away for me.

The moment will come when you, the caregiver, will say to yourself, "I need help!" Whether that moment is the result of a sudden call from the emergency room or is reached after prolonged eldercaring, it may be a moment of panic. The encouraging news, however, is that you are not alone and there IS help available. Along with an aging population has come an increase in the number and accessibility of services for the elderly. With a little patience and perseverance, you should be able to find the optimal mix of services to meet your current needs.

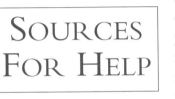

START CLOSE TO HOME

Begin your search for help in the most obvious places — with those closest to your elder such as family, friends and neighbors. Your elder's doctor(s) will provide not only information about medical needs, but will also be an important link to Medicare and other health insurance plans. Continue your search by looking at the surrounding community, including churches, local government, social services and agencies on aging. Finally, invaluable information is available from national support groups for the elderly, national organizations for specific diseases and federal government agencies.

While family and friends will continue to be a source of help and support, neighbors are an often overlooked resource. In many communities there are high concentrations of seniors who have "aged in place" forming what are referred

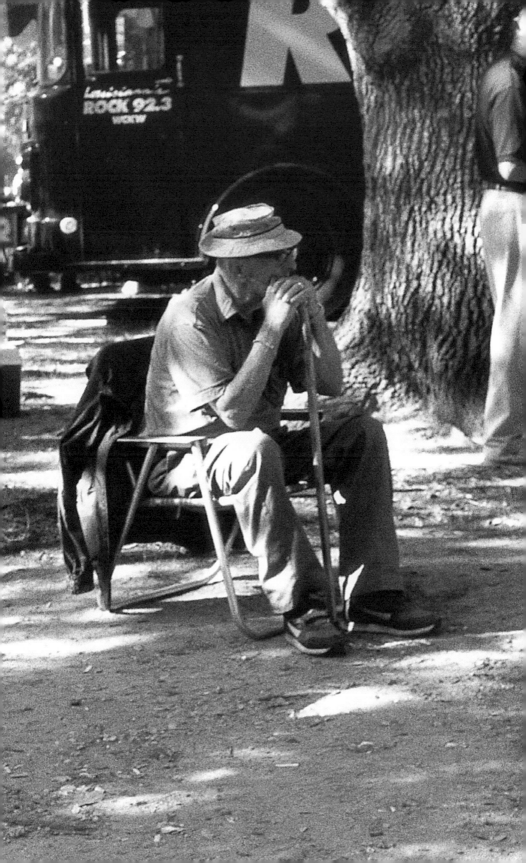

to as NORCs (naturally occurring retirement communities). NORCs, as opposed to planned retirement communities, simply evolve on their own. Many neighbors give informal support to each other, whether simply by calling to check on each other's well-being or by running errands for those unable to leave home. The existence of NORCs also provides the opportunity for sharing of professional health care or other services. Although service providers often have minimum time requirements for housecalls, many flexible providers are now willing to break up the typical four hour minimum among groups of citizens living in NORCs. For instance, a senior may only need brief periods of assistance with such activities as bathing and dressing in order to live independently. The NORCs provide

access to services which might not otherwise be affordable.

Medicare is the primary health insurance provider and the most important health care resource for the majority of those 65 and older in the United States. Medicare coverage will influence many of your decisions regarding health care services and your choice of providers. Careful consultation with your elder's primary doctor(s) should help to establish the best combination of services. It is very important to obtain a copy of the Medicare pamphlet outlining the services and durable medical equipment (walkers, wheelchairs, etc.) which are covered. Also be sure to refer to a list of Medicare-approved home health care providers in your senior's area.

You may want to consider other sources of health care coverage and

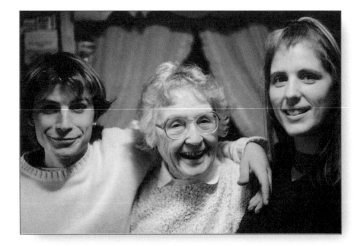

N o t e s

_____

_____

_____

_____

_____

_____

_____

_____

_____

_____

_____

_____

_____

_____

_____

_____

_____

_____

compare them to that offered by Medicare in order to determine the best overall care affordable to your elder. Supplemental health insurance may well be worth the extra expense, particularly those policies which cover prescription medicines, home care and nursing home care.

Social workers have current knowledge of services and programs that are available in the local community. Many of these services are available on a sliding fee schedule, rather than being limited to those who qualify for welfare. If your elder has been hospitalized, she should be assisted by a hospital social worker in finding a local nursing home bed or ensuring that home health support is in place.

Local churches and other volunteer organizations provide services, such as daily telephone calls to check on the elderly or running errands to the grocery or druggist. Meals-on-Wheels provides food and support to the home-bound in many communities, and the local Agency on Aging and Long-term Care Ombudsman may be valuable sources of information. New sources for help are continually being developed.

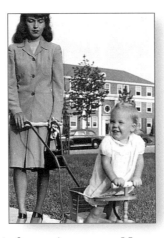

FEDERAL AGENCIES

ADMINISTRATION ON AGING. *Leading advocate within federal government for older Americans. Funds state and area agencies, research, demonstration and training programs.* 202-619-0724 or 202-401-4541. www.aoa.gov

DEPARTMENT OF HEALTH AND HUMAN SERVICES. www.os.dhhs.gov **HEALTH CARE FINANCING ADMINISTRATION.** *HCFA administers Medicare and Medicaid programs, offers free publications and operates a telephone hot line/information service.* HCFA, 7500 Security Blvd., Baltimore, MD 21244-1850. 410-786-3000. HCFA Medicare Hotline 800-638-6833. www.hcfa.gov

MEDICARE. *Provides basic protection for hospital care (Part A) and supple-mental protection for additional medical costs (Part B). Available to those 65 or older or those who receive Social Security disability payments. Call for eligibility requirements.* Part A 800-655-1636. Part B 800-444-4606. See Health Care Financing Administration.

NATIONAL INSTITUTE ON AGING. *NIA conducts and supports studies of Alzheimer's Disease and related dementia, aging, frailty, disability and rehabilitation, health and effective functioning, long-term care and other special problems and needs of older people.* NIA Alzheimer's Disease Education and Referral Center, P.O. Box 8250, Silver Spring, MD 20907-8250. 800-438-4380. www.alzheimers.org

NATIONAL INSTITUTES OF HEALTH. *The National Institute on Aging is part of NIH. NIH is an excellent source of information about specific diseases.* www.nih.gov

PENSION AND WELFARE BENEFITS ADMINISTRATION. www.dol. gov/dol/pwba

PENSION BENEFIT GUARANTY CORPORATION. www.pbgc.gov

SOCIAL SECURITY ADMINISTRATION. Information 800-772-1213. www.ssa.gov

Notes

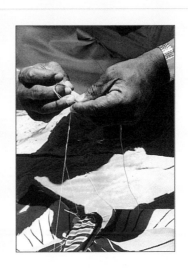

VETERANS ADMINISTRATION. 6401 Security Blvd., Baltimore, MD 21235, www.va.gov

ASSOCIATIONS AND FOUNDATIONS

ALLIANCE FOR AGING RESEARCH. *Independent nonprofit organization founded to promote medical research. Pamphlets available.* 2021 K St., NW, Washington, DC 20006, 202-293-2856.

ALZHEIMER'S ASSOCIATION. *Provides information and referrals to local chapters, which in turn refer people to local services and support groups. Helpful to families dealing with other forms of dementia as well.* 919 N. Michigan Ave., Suite 1000, Chicago IL 60611, 800-272-3900.

AMERICAN ASSOCIATION OF RETIRED PERSONS. *This is the largest non-profit organization devoted to meeting the needs of older Americans.*

Notes

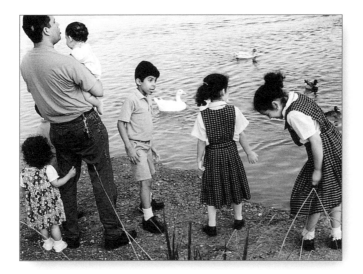

Publications are available on legal, financial, insurance and care giving topics. 1909 K St., NW, Washington, DC 20049, 202-434-2277 in the Washington, DC area 800-424-3410 outside of Washington. www.aarp.org

AMERICAN HEALTH ASSISTANCE FOUNDATION. *Nonprofit organization dedicated to funding research on age-related and degenerative diseases, educating the public about them, and offering emergency financial assistance to Alzheimer's patients and their caregivers.* 15825 Shady Grove Road, Suite 140, Rockville, MD 20850, 800-437-2423.

AMERICAN HEALTH CARE ASSOCIATION. *Represents 11,000 nonprofit and for-profit nursing facilities assisted living and subacute providers nationally. Provides helpful information* about choosing a care facility. 202-842-4444.

AMERICAN HEART ASSOCIATION. *Call for referrals to local chapters which have information on stroke and support groups.* 7272 Greenville Ave., Dallas, TX 75231, 800-242-1793.

AMERICAN PARKINSON'S DISEASE ASSOCIATION. *Sends out general information and links people to local APDA centers.* 60 Bay St., Room 401, Staten Island, NY 10301, 800-223-2732.

ASSISTED LIVING FEDERATION OF AMERICA. *Offers free information and national referral services plus a 15–page consumer guide.* 703-691-8100.

CHILDREN OF AGING PARENTS. *This is a national clearinghouse for caregivers and professionals, offering referrals, educational programs and support groups.* 1609 Woodbourne Road, Suite 302A, Levittown, PA 19057-1151.

Eldercare Locator. *A good place to start when looking for local services.* 800-677-1116.

Family Caregiver Alliance. *Information clearinghouse for people caring for someone with stroke or other cognitive impairment.* 425 Bush St. Suite 500, San Francisco, CA 94108, 415-434-3388.

Hospice. *A medically directed, team-oriented program of care for terminally ill patients. The hospice mission is to treat the physical, emotional and spiritual needs of the patient. Family members are an essential component of the care giving team, and hospices often offering bereavement groups and other support programs for families.* National Hospice Helpline 800-658-8898. HospiceLink, 800-331-1620.

National Alliance of Senior Citizens. *Membership fee, but benefits include insurance and phone discounts.* 202-986-0117.

National Association of Area Agencies on Aging. *Makes referrals to local agencies on aging and co-sponsors Eldercare Locator, a toll-free telephone databank of nationwide community services for older people, including health, homemaker, nutrition, transporta-*

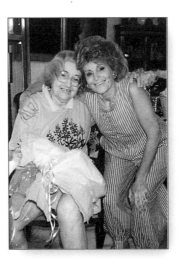

tion, legal and other services. 202-296-8130.

National Association for Continence. *A nonprofit organization that has brochures, books, videos and tapes giving information about incontinence. Has catalogues for special products and doctors who specialize in incontinence.* P.O. Box 544, Union, SC 29379, 800-252-3337.

National Association for Home Care. *On request will send information on tips for choosing a home-care agency.* 228 7th St., SE, Washington, DC 20003, 202-547-7424.

National Federation of Inter-faith Volunteer Caregivers. 368 Broadway, Suite 103, Kingston, NY 12401, 800-350-7438.

National Caregiving Foundation. *Helps caregivers of people with life-threatening and catastrophic illnesses.* 801 N. Pitt St., #116, Alexandria, VA 22314. 703-299-9300. To order a Caregivers Support Kit, call 800-930-1357.

National Caucus & Center on Black Aged. *National interracial membership organization works to improve living conditions for low-income*

Notes

_____
_____
_____
_____
_____
_____
_____
_____
_____
_____
_____
_____
_____
_____
_____
_____
_____
_____
_____
_____

and minority older persons. Membership fee. 202-637-8400.

NATIONAL CITIZENS' COALI-TIONS FOR NURSING HOME REFORM. *Works to improve the quality of care and life in nursing homes and other long-term care facilities. Provides free fact sheets and offers resource refer-* *rals.* 202-332-2275.

NATIONAL COUNCIL OF SENIOR CITIZENS. *Political activities related to the elderly and sponsors workshops, maintains a library and operates housing assistance and other programs. Membership fee required.* 301-578-8800.

National Family Care-givers Association. *Offers assistance to those caring for a loved one who is chronically ill or disabled as well as information, support and referrals. Resource guide available. Membership fee.* 800-896-3650.

National Meals on Wheels Foundation. *Makes referrals to local meal delivery programs and congregate or group dining programs.* 2675 44th St. SW Suite 305, Grand Rapids, MI 49509, 800-999-6262.

Ombudsman Programs. *Protects the rights of people in nursing homes and community residences. Call Area Agencies on Aging.*

The Lighthouse National Center for Vision and Aging. *Information on every aspect of vision loss and eye disease, as well as for referrals to state agencies, local services, support groups and low-vision centers.* 111 East 59th St., New York, NY 10022, 212-821-9200, 800-334-5497.

United Seniors Health Cooperative. *Gives guidance on long-term care insurance, housing alternatives, financial assistance and other resources. "Open membership," by contributions.* 202-479-6973.

Visiting Nurse Associations of America. *A national coalition of nonprofit, community-based home health care providers.* 800-426-2547.

Well Spouse Foundation. *A national network offering local support groups, education, and advocacy for issues affecting the elderly. A newsletter, "Mainstay," focuses on the problems of caring for a chronically ill partner.* P.O. Box 10023, New York, NY 10023. 212-644-1241 or 800-838-0879.

Companies That Offer Specialized Equipment

AT&T Special Needs. *Telephone accessories for those with special needs.* 800-833-3232.

Centex Life Solutions— The Life Improvement Store. 703-532-6800.

Lifeline. *Provides emergency response for those with medical problems.* 800-642-0045.

Medic Alert Bracelet. *Identi-fying bracelets containing name, address, phone number and diagnosis.* 800-432-5378.

Sears Home Health Care Specialogue. *Home health care products for the disabled.* 800-326-1750.

Tubular Specialists. *Grab bars for tub & walls.* 800-421-2961.

Yellow Pages. *Check your phone book for other medical suppliers in your area.*

N o t e s

_____

_____

_____

_____

Use this journal to
keep track of new
companies and
sources.

_____

_____

_____

_____

_____

_____

_____

_____

_____

_____

_____

_____

_____

_____

_____

_____

_____

_____

_____

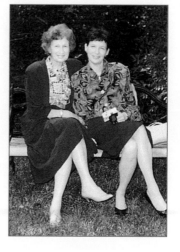

_____

_____

_____

_____

_____

VITAL INFORMATION AND ELDERCARING PLANNER

*T*his *vital information and note sections are provided so that you can keep up with the day-to-day necessities of eldercaring. Use them to record appointments, calls that need to be made, care giving errands and obligations, health related developments and special occasions to remember. Doing this will help you to keep focused and organized … more important than ever now that you are managing your own life as well as that of another. By putting your plans down on paper, you will not be stressed by so many frantic, last-minute situations, by the inability to answer physicians' questions or by forgotten commitments. It will make you feel more in control of care giving and more in control of your own life.*

If you are reluctant to put financial information into the journal, duplicate the forms, fill in the information, and keep them somewhere safe and easy to access.

❤ **TIPS FOR DEALING WITH THE MEDICAL PROFESSION**

❤ Write down questions before medical appointments.

❤ Write to the doctor ahead of time with questions. This allows the doctor to think about answers and also to use them as background in dealing with your elder during the appointment.

❤ Keep track of questions you wish you had asked the doctor!

❤ Take notes while in the doctor's office.

❤ Take the following to medical appointments:

1. List of current (including "over-the-counter") medicines

2. List of past medications and whether they were successful or not

3. List of allergies

4. Copies of the patient's medical history, along with names and phone numbers of previous doctors

5. Copies of family medical history

6. Descriptions of current problem and symptoms.

❤ Let the patient answer the questions so the doctor can observe how he responds. Allow the doctor and patient to develop a rapport. You can always provide corrections and more details later.

♥ Keep extra copies of medical documents (insurance, Medicare, Medicaid).

♥ Inform doctors of any difficulties your elder is facing in daily living. They may have solutions.

♥ Be sure that medical professionals keep in touch and are aware of each other's treatments. Your pharmacist can help with this!

Be careful with this information!! Guard it like a credit card.

VITAL INFORMATION

NAME(S) _____

ADDRESS _____

_____

PHONE _____

LANDLORD _____

PHONE _____

NEIGHBOR _____

PHONE _____

ADDRESS _____

_____

NEIGHBOR _____

PHONE _____

ADDRESS _____

_____

FRIEND _____

PHONE _____

ADDRESS _____

_____

FRIEND _____

PHONE _____

ADDRESS _____

FAMILY MEMBERS & PHONE NUMBERS

NAME _____

RELATIONSHIP _____

ADDRESS _____

PHONE (HOME) _____(OFFICE) _____

NAME _____

RELATIONSHIP _____

ADDRESS _____

PHONE (HOME) _____(OFFICE) _____

NAME _____

RELATIONSHIP _____

ADDRESS _____

PHONE (HOME) _____(OFFICE) _____

NAME _____

RELATIONSHIP _____

ADDRESS _____

PHONE (HOME) _____(OFFICE) _____

NAME _____

RELATIONSHIP _____

ADDRESS _____

PHONE (HOME) _____(OFFICE) _____

EMERGENCY NUMBERS

FIRE _____

POLICE/SHERIFF _____

AMBULANCE _____

BLOOD TYPE _____

AUTOMOBILE/TRANSPORTATION

AUTO MAKE & LICENSE NO. _____

_____

_____

DRIVERS LICENSE _____

EXPIRATION _____

SPOUSES DRIVERS LICENSE _____

EXPIRATION _____

AUTOMOBILE INSURANCE AGENT _____

ADDRESS _____

PHONE _____

POLICY NUMBER _____

ROAD SERVICE POLICY NUMBER _____

PHONE _____

TRANSPORTATION/TAXI SERVICE(S) _____

_____

_____

_____

_____

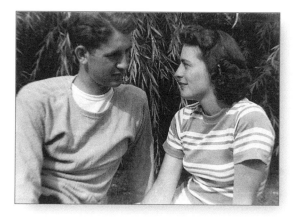

MEDICAL NUMBERS

DOCTOR _____

PHONE _____

ADDRESS _____

DOCTOR _____

PHONE _____

ADDRESS _____

NURSING AGENCY _____

PHONE _____

ADDRESS _____

CLINIC _____

PHONE _____

ADDRESS _____

HOSPITAL _____

PHONE _____

ADDRESS _____

ALLERGIES _____

_____

_____

_____

_____

_____

MEDICATIONS & DOSAGES _____

_____

_____

_____

_____

_____

MEDICAL INSURANCE _____

PHONE _____

POLICY NUMBER _____

ADDRESS _____

SUPPLEMENTAL MEDICAL INSURANCE _____

_____

PHONE _____

POLICY NUMBER _____

ADDRESS _____

PHARMACIST_____

PHONE_____

ADDRESS _____

DENTIST _____

PHONE _____

ADDRESS _____

DENTAL INSURANCE _____

PHONE _____

POLICY NUMBER _____

ADDRESS _____

OPTOMETRIST _____

PHONE _____

ADDRESS _____

VETERINARIAN _____

PHONE _____

ADDRESS _____

FINANCIAL INFORMATION
(Sample Form)

SOCIAL SECURITY NUMBER _____

DATE & PLACE OF BIRTH _____

_____

SPOUSE'S SOCIAL SECURITY NUMBER _____

SPOUSE'S DATE & PLACE OF BIRTH _____

_____

BANK _____

PHONE_____

ADDRESS_____

ACCOUNT NUMBERS _____

_____

BANK _____

PHONE _____

ADDRESS _____

ACCOUNT NUMBERS _____

_____

BANK _____

PHONE _____

ADDRESS _____

ACCOUNT NUMBERS _____

_____

SAFE-DEPOSIT BOX LOCATION _____

_____

ACCOUNTANT/FINANCIAL PLANNER _____

PHONE _____

ADDRESS _____

ATTORNEY _____

PHONE _____

ADDRESS _____

HOMEOWNERS INSURANCE _____

POLICY NUMBER _____

PHONE _____

ADDRESS _____

LIFE INSURANCE COMPANY _____

POLICY NUMBER _____

PHONE _____

ADDRESS _____

CHARGE ACCOUNTS & CREDIT CARDS _____

_____

_____

_____

_____

_____

_____

_____

_____

_____

MISCELLANEOUS _____

_____

_____

_____

_____

_____

_____

_____

_____

_____

_____

PROFESSIONAL HELPERS

EMPLOYEES (home aide, housekeeping, yard work) & phone numbers

_____

_____

_____

_____

REPAIRMEN (car, furnace, appliances, plumber, electrician) & phone numbers

_____

_____

_____

_____

PET SITTER _____

PHONE _____

ADDRESS _____

UTILITIES AND SERVICES

WATER COMPANY _____

GAS COMPANY _____

ELECTRIC COMPANY _____

TELEPHONE COMPANY _____

LONG DISTANCE COMPANY _____

LOCKSMITH _____

CABLE COMPANY _____

HOUSE ALARM COMPANY _____

SOCIAL INFORMATION

ACTIVITIES/LOCATIONS/DAYS/PHONE NUMBERS
(Senior Center, Clubs, Classes)

_____

_____

_____

CHURCH/SYNAGOGUE _____

CLERGYMAN _____

PHONE _____

NEWSPAPER/MAGAZINE SUBSCRIPTIONS _____

_____

_____

_____

_____

_____

_____

HOME DELIVERED MEALS _____

_____

_____

_____

_____

_____

_____

GROCERY STORES THAT DELIVER _____

_____

_____

_____

_____

_____

_____

RESTAURANTS THAT DELIVER _____

_____

_____

_____

_____

_____

_____

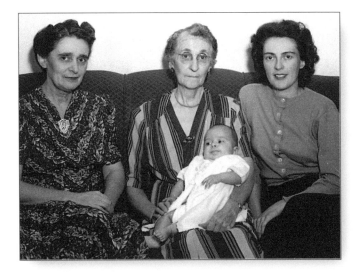

Notes

Notes

> "Never let a problem
> to be solved become
> more important than
> a person to be loved."
>
> — Barbara Johnson,
> *The Joy Journal*

WHEN YOU NEED A FRIEND

For the Fourteen Friends, the greatest benefit from this book has been the continual inspiration we've received from sharing each other's experiences. Since we started writing this book, it has become even more obvious to us that eldercaring needs change daily. Our loved ones have moved to assisted care and nursing homes, and there have been several deaths. We have shared practical solutions to every conceivable scenario. Throughout, the continued support and camaraderie within our group have eased the emotional stress of these transitions.

Friends and acquaintances who knew we were writing this book have often mentioned their personal need for a guide like this. Knowing of our interest and concern for this subject has encouraged them to share their own situations, difficulties, and successes. We thank them for giving us the confidence to proceed.

We hope that as you read this book and record your own thoughts and solutions, you will feel like the fifteenth friend in our group. Just as our friendships are stronger as a result of sharing, we hope that you too will gain strength from this book and from your own support groups. We hope that these ideas will help you develop a closer relationship with those for whom you care.

BOOKS THAT WERE HELPFUL TO US

Care giving — How to Care for Your Elderly Mother and Stay Sane, by E. Jane Mall (New York: Ballantine Books, 1990).

Helping Yourself Help Others: A Book for Caregivers, by Rosalynn Carter with Susan K. Golant (New York: Times Books, 1994).

How Did I Become My Parent's Parent, by Harriet Sarnoff Schiff (New York: Penguin Books, 1996).

How to Care for Aging Parents, by Virginia Morris (New York: Workman Publishing Company, Inc., 1996).

The Complete Eldercare Planner, by Joy Loverde (Silvercare Productions, 1993, reprinted 1997 by Joy Loverde).

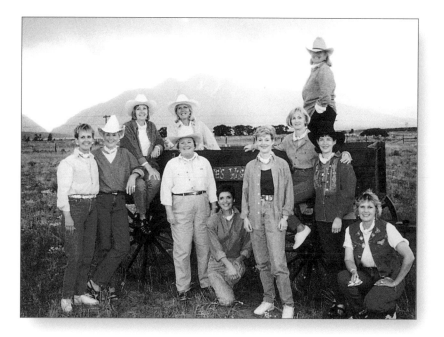

A SPECIAL NOTE OF THANKS

Fourteen Friends thank their families & friends for their support and encouragement in the writing of this book. To our parents, in-laws, grandparents and others, we thank you for the chance to give back to you and the opportunity to share. We especially thank our immediate families, husbands and significant others for their patience, love and interest while we were so involved in our book. We thank our agent, Rue Judd, for her confidence, enthusiasm and guidance. We appreciate the support and professionalism of our publisher, Kathleen Hughes, and our graphic designer, Caroline Brock. We're most thankful that our friendships have gotten even stronger during the creation of *Fourteen Friends Guide to Eldercaring.*

Share your ideas and suggestions for eldercaring with your friends. Write to us at:

Fourteen Friends
c/o Capital Books
P.O. Box 605
Herndon, Virginia
20172-0605
F14Friends@aol.com

INDEX